INTENSERCISE

Tapping the Forgotten Secret to Multiplying Your Workout Results

Specifically Designed for the 40+ Exerciser

By
Andrew Kilikauskas
and
Michelle Kilikauskas, RKC

Train hard, train smart and NEVER quit!

Published by:
Mojave Gems, Ridgecrest, CA
Website: www.intensercise.com

ISBN: 978-0-9853076-0-8
First edition published October 2012

Photographs by Andrew Kilikauskas and Michelle Kilikauskas
Illustrations by Robbie Short
Cover Design by Chris Di Natale
Interior Design and Layout by Marian Hartsough
Editing by Barbara Ardinger

Publishers Cataloging-in-Publication Data

Kilikauskas, Andrew and Kilikauskas, Michelle
Intensercise / Andrew Kilikauskas and Michelle Kilikauskas
        p.   cm.
Includes bibliographical references and index.
ISBN: 978-0-9853076-0-8
1. Exercise 2. Physical Fitness 3. Kettlebells 4. Cardiovascular Fitness 5. Weight Training
613.71

Disclaimers

We've made every effort to convey that when training for strength and conditioning safety is always important. It's important to remember to proceed slowly and with caution. Get help when needed.

The bottom line is that you proceed at your own risk. Your body is your responsibility, so look after it.

All medical experts agree that you should consult a physician before starting any physical training program.

We get specific about exercise equipment in this book. We recommend products that we have personal experience with and think work well. We have received no money, discounts, or any other compensation or inducements to mention any product.

Contents

Chapter 3

Conditioning Part 1 – Cardiovascular Capacity (VO2 Max) and Aerobic Capacity (Lactate Threshold)   43

Chapter 4
Conditioning, Part 2 — Muscular Endurance 65

Chapter 5
Putting Strength and Conditioning Together 85

Chapter 6

Recovery – the Other Crucial Factor   103

Chapter 7

Diet and Supplements Are Important, Too   113

Chapter 11
Finding Your Own Way to Extraordinary Fitness 155

Afterword
Final Thoughts on Staying Fit in Real Life 161

Glossary 165

Bibliography 169

Index 173

Introduction

If you're reading this book with the hope of learning how to achieve extraordinary fitness in three easy twenty-minute workouts a week, stop right now. Put this book down and go back to the couch in front of your big screen HDTV where infomercials will keep feeding your fantasy.

If, however, you're ready to leave fantasy behind and embrace reality, this book will give you practical knowledge and information that will enable you to greatly increase your conditioning and level of strength. Whether you're a serious athlete or a weekend warrior or just someone who wants to get and stay in great shape, this book can show you how to achieve a significantly higher level of overall fitness.

You'll need to add some equipment, a lot of serious, focused effort, and a consistent commitment of time. The combination of knowledge, tools, time, and action will produce powerful results.

The how-to template presented in this book gives you a results-driven exercise routine that will increase your levels of strength and conditioning. This greater fitness can then be used for enjoyment-driven recreational or sports activities. The program also has the substantial side benefits of improving your health and functionality in all areas of your life. We provide specific recommendations in all aspects of this program that you can start to use immediately.

What kind of results can you expect? First, you'll get strong. You'll be able to carry 50-pound bags of fertilizer around your garden without strain. Or haul those full kegs of beer and ice-filled coolers out to your pool for that Fourth of July BBQ. Or stack bales of hay for your horses. Whether you're a serious or a recreational athlete, greater strength will improve your performance as you play basketball, climb rocks, ski, or participate in any other sport you choose. As a side effect of this kind of strength, your muscles will be hard and toned, not flabby.

Second, you'll develop your entire cardiovascular system (heart, lungs, and circulatory system) and increase its capacity and endurance. You'll be able to go out hiking for an entire day to bag a local mountain peak, and if you're still on the trail when it's starting to get dark, you'll be able to hike faster back down the hill and get to your car before it gets too dark to see the trail. You're able to go fast when you need or want to. (It's always fun to set such a torrid pace that your companions are forced to beg you to slow down.) The side effect of excellent aerobic conditioning is improved health, especially improved cardiovascular health. This is something that's pretty important to everyone, especially for those of us in middle age or beyond.

Third, those newly strong muscles will develop the endurance to keep going and going and going. You'll think nothing of spending two eight-hour days over a weekend digging a koi pond with a pick and shovel. The side effect of great muscular endurance is a body with larger muscles and much less fat.

It's all about basic strength and conditioning. This means increasing your body's strength, cardiovascular endurance, and muscular endurance capabilities. Strength and conditioning, also referred to as fitness, give you the ability to do so much more physically. Fitness improves your overall health, too. Basic strength and conditioning provide the base upon which you build so that you can pursue all kinds of physical activities from hiking to rock climbing to bicycling to kayaking to skiing to anything that you want to do. If you want to be and stay active, strength and conditioning will give you the capability to do so. Strength and conditioning let you do whatever you want to do—sports, activities, travel.

Why listen to us about improving your strength and conditioning? Because we've been there. We've been on a decades-long journey to live an active life and be able to continue to do so as we grow older.

Both of us are average physical specimens, and we're mostly average in the many sports we've participated in, the exception being Michelle's excellence in powerlifting. We've tried lots of methods of getting and staying fit. Some things worked, some didn't. When a method didn't work, we abandoned it. If something did work, we pursued it further and kept using it.

This means we're speaking from years and years of research and trial and error investigation into what works for average people to increase their strength, cardio endurance, and muscular endurance.

We've worked with and learned from top coaches in weightlifting, bicycling, and kettlebell lifting. And we've rubbed shoulders with elite athletes and talked with them about what worked for them to improve their strength and conditioning as well as excel in their sport.

We've also subjected various exercise methods to hard numerical evaluation. Did a method make us stronger? We evaluated it by noting if we were able to lift heavier weights or not. Did a method increase our cardio endurance? We evaluated it by noting if the training increased our power at VO2 max, which is a measurement of the maximum amount (volume) of oxygen that your body's cardiovascular system can take in and process. In other words, it's the capability of your cardiovascular system. It's the "gold standard" measurement of your cardiovascular fitness. Did a method increase our muscular endurance? We measured how much longer we were able to swing, snatch, or clean and jerk a kettlebell than before.

By now, we've found methods that really work for the average person to develop and maintain high levels of strength and conditioning. We believe that they will work equally well for elite athletes and not-so-elite athletes.

The core principles of our training techniques and programs

Over the years we've tried all sorts of training techniques and programs. Some were basic and straightforward, others complex. In our experience, simple is almost always better. There are two rules we use to evaluate different training techniques and programs.

First, we apply the Occam's razor principle, which is that, all else being equal, the simplest method of achieving a goal is the best. For example, if the goal is to do more chin-ups, the simplest way is to do a lot of chin-ups. More complex programs using lots of other exercises like lat pull downs, barbell rows, cable rows, etc., and using different repetition patterns are very hard to implement and tend to be much more time consuming and much less effective than the direct approach.

Second, we follow the 80/20 rule: eighty percent of the results come from twenty percent of the effort. Identify that critical twenty percent, and even the most time-pressed boomer can achieve amazing results. Another example comes from the world of strength. If you focus all your effort on only two exercises, a big pull and a press, you can achieve eighty percent or more of your strength potential. Cutting out other exercises gives you the most bang for your effort and simplifies the whole process (see Occam's razor, above).

Note that simple and focused can be much more effective and efficient than trying everything you see in an ad or infomercial or read in a fitness magazine, but it's not necessarily easy. *You must put in the work.* Achieving extraordinary fitness also takes time. There's no way around that. How much time? Plan on four to eight hours a week. Less than four hours can work if you're just starting out or if you're just maintaining your current condition because you're pressed for time for some reason. But less than four hours just isn't enough time to do what you need to do to improve your fitness. It's OK for maintenance, but it won't give you significant improvement.

If your goal is to establish and maintain a solid level of fitness, then you just don't need more than about eight hours a week. If you're putting in more than eight hours a week, you're exercising for fun or training to seriously compete in a sport. That isn't a bad thing. We encourage you to have fun with and enjoy your strength and conditioning training. And it's great to find and participate in a sport you enjoy. It's just that you don't have to put in that much time to reach and stay at a very high level of overall fitness.

Four to eight hours a week sounds like a lot to most sedentary Americans, so let's get some perspective. It's only a fraction of the 168 hours in a week. It's also a lot less than the 40+ hours a week almost everyone puts in at work. Or, for that matter, the much longer work weeks many modern professionals and entrepreneurs put in.

> We're going focus on the twenty percent of work that'll produce eighty percent of the benefits.

But maybe you think it's not possible to get really fit in only four to eight hours a week. For example, many recreational triathletes feel the need to work out twice as much. Or more! It's probably true that they're fitter than if they only exercised four to eight hours a week, but they're definitely at the point of diminishing returns, doing eighty percent more work to get the last twenty percent of the results.

We're going focus on the twenty percent of work that'll produce eighty percent of the benefits.

If you truly are a competitive athlete, then you will have to train more. You will have to put in many hours a week practicing your sport on top of your strength and conditioning training. You will also want to have higher levels of strength and conditioning, which will take more time and effort. Our point is that achieving and maintaining a solid level of fitness doesn't require more time.

And the reality is that few of us have the time or inclination to pursue much more than four to eight hours a week of physical training. Up to about an hour a day strikes us as reasonable and doable, but stretch that out to two or more hours a day, and we balk. An hour a day of physical exercise is a serious commitment, but one that is within reach for almost everyone. Most people could cut out an hour of TV watching or Internet surfing. If we reorder our priorities and perhaps let go of some other things (some of which we may also think are important), then we can find an hour a day. Almost everyone can do this.

As important as the psychological issue is the fact that very few older trainees can handle more than this volume of work, recover from it, and continue to improve instead of regressing. Every older athlete has noticed this fact of life: while they can still train intensely, they can't handle the same volume of work that they could when they were younger.

Four to eight hours a week appears to be the "sweet spot." It's enough time to build and maintain extraordinary fitness, and it's also a reasonable and doable amount. This is the time commitment that you will have to make.

Use the right equipment

To achieve the results you want, you'll need some equipment. The good news is that, generally speaking, the necessary tools are few, and affordable. An Olympic barbell set, two or three different size kettlebells, and a stopwatch or timer are all you need for strength and muscular endurance training. For cardio endurance training, you'll need a bicycle, a power meter with heart rate monitor, and an indoor trainer for your bicycle. Used intelligently and diligently, that's the basic equipment you'll need.

For more details about the right equipment, including what features to look for and what it might cost, you can skip forward to Chapter 9. There you will also find information about useful accessories that will make training more efficient and/or comfortable.

Since you don't need any fancy exercise machines, you can forgo that expensive gym membership. Instead, work out more conveniently and with greater focus in your garage, basement, yard, or outdoors on the road or trail whenever you want to. It's what you do with the tools that produces results, not the tools themselves.

Gyms can be handy and motivating, but mostly they're just showrooms for fancy exercise machines and gathering places for people who are just going through the motions of what they "should" do. Gyms are full of distractions, both social and technological, and although serious trainees can use a gym in a pinch, it isn't your best choice. Instead of paying for an expensive gym membership, consider using the cash to invest in your own equipment.

By exercising at home with your own equipment, you can not only save the commute time to and from the gym, but you can also focus on the important tasks at hand. Plus, when the tools are in your garage or basement, you'll have no excuses not to use them. As for motivation, we've found that lasting motivation comes from within, not from other people. No gym environment can substitute for real desire to improve yourself physically.

By exercising at home with your own equipment, you can not only save the commute time to and from the gym, but you can also focus on the important tasks at hand. Plus, when the tools are in your garage or basement, you'll have no excuses not to use them. As for motivation, we've found that lasting motivation comes from within, not from other people. No gym environment can substitute for real desire to improve yourself physically.

We've found that old-school basics like barbells and kettlebells work amazingly well when compared to some of the newer weight training machines and gadgets. At the same time, when new technology works better than older tools, we adopt it readily. One example of technology that truly works is the power meter with heart rate monitor. Its feedback makes it much easier to do cardio training effectively and efficiently.

While both low tech and high tech equipment can be effective and helpful, it's important to remember that the tools should never be the focus. Focus on the work you're doing. Focus on using the equipment intelligently, consistently, and with intensity.

Bottom line, you will need to acquire some equipment. You'll find that the right equipment is worth the price you pay to buy good stuff. There is no alternative. You need good equipment to achieve extraordinary fitness.

Motivation

Your final requirement is serious, focused effort. Once you've laid out what you need to do clearly and in writing to achieve your goals, you then need to actually *do the work*. Sometimes it will be hard. You will be working your muscles beyond their comfort zone. They'll get sore. You'll sweat. You'll breathe hard. Your heart will pound. You'll wonder why you're doing this to yourself.

That's when you'll need to have a reason for doing all this hard work. A reason that's important to you. A reason that motivates you.

Perhaps you're doing it because you don't want to be a middle aged, fat guy whose belly hangs over his belt while he's driving his red Mercedes convertible. You want to stand out. You want to be an extraordinary physical specimen who doesn't need to compensate. Or perhaps you're doing it because you want to feel confident wearing a bikini on the beach. Satisfying one's ego can be a powerful motivation.

> Once you've laid out what you need to do clearly and in writing to achieve your goals, you then need to actually *do the work*. Sometimes it will be hard. You will be working your muscles beyond their comfort zone. They'll get sore. You'll sweat. You'll breathe hard. Your heart will pound. You'll wonder why you're doing this to yourself.

Or perhaps you're more practical. You want to get rid of those nagging aches and pains that seem to get more numerous and troublesome every year. Or you want to be physically able to do the things you want to do, whether that's working in your garden or trekking to Machu Picchu.

Whatever your motivation, you need to make it clear to yourself. And you need to remind yourself often. Consistency, sticking with it—that's a big part of serious effort.

By the way, being middle-aged is no barrier to achieving extraordinary fitness. The human body responds to physical stimulus at any age, from 20 to 50 to 70. If you exercise and eat right, you'll improve your fitness no matter what your current condition may be. Whether you've kept

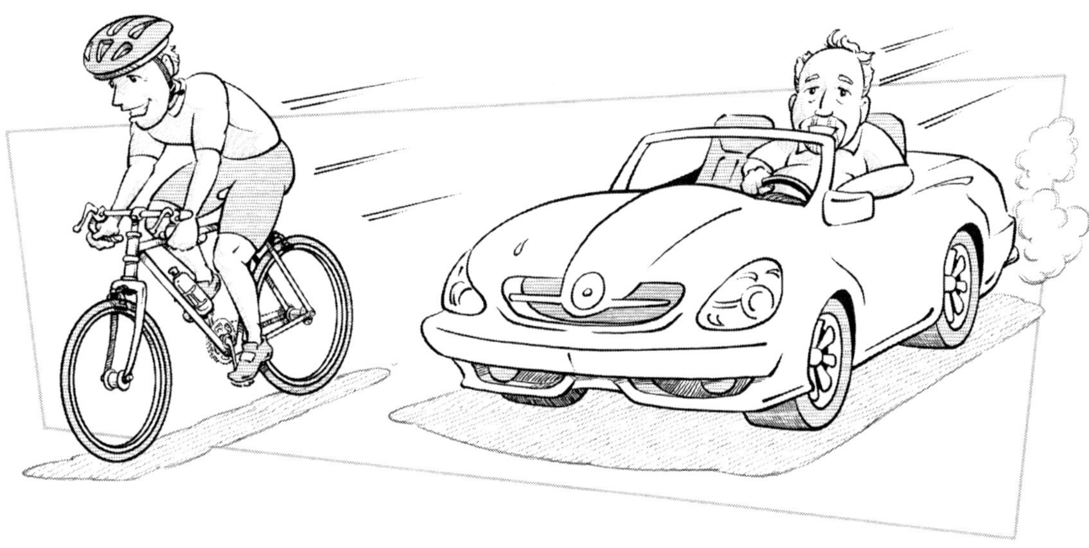

Life is about choices.

active and in pretty good shape over the years or you've neglected your body, you can improve physically. It's truly never too late to start. Accumulated wear and tear over the years does play into the ultimate level of fitness you can achieve, but no matter where you start, you can improve.

If you're a bit older and you've let yourself go to pot, there's actually good news. When you start to exercise, you will make dramatic and speedy progress. Your previously neglected body will visibly improve, week by week. The bad news, of course, is that you have a lot further to go to reach excellent fitness. The math is cruel. If you're 50 and in half as good condition as you

> Consistency, sticking with it—that's a big part of serious effort.

were at age 25, you will need to improve 100 percent to just equal your condition at age 25. To improve on it will take more than a hundred percent. Hard, yes, but it can be done with consistent effort and patience. But even if you never do exceed your fitness at a younger age, the improvements in fitness you do make will manifest themselves in very noticeable improvements in the quality of your life.

On the other hand, if you've kept yourself in decent shape over the years, you'll face different challenges. You can also improve significantly, but your progress will be slower and often not immediately obvious. Also, you'll need to revamp your training program. This can be hard to do, especially if you've been following it for many years. The good news is that you don't have nearly as far to go to reach truly extraordinary fitness.

Now you might not believe that anyone could be in better shape in middle age than when they were in their twenties. Especially if they were athletic in high school and college. But it's a fact. In cycling there are many over-50 masters riders that are riding faster times in standard

40-kilometer (24.8 mile) time trials than when they were in their twenties and thirties. The same applies to master powerlifters who continue to improve into their forties and fifties. A famous example is Olympic swimmer Dara Torres. She was swimming faster times in her forties than she did in her twenties.

This kind of progress has been made possible by improved training methods based on science, not tradition, on better equipment, better diet and supplements, and on improved recovery methods like massage. Believe it. *Age is not a barrier to physical improvement.*

Here's the bottom line. You can develop your body's strength and endurance capabilities to a very high level. Application of the practical knowledge in this book will enable you to achieve this. If you combine that knowledge with basic equipment, the appropriate amount of time, and focused effort, you'll increase your fitness. You will be able to go further than you now think you can. Maybe even further than you imagine in your dreams.

What about us?

When Michelle was in elementary and high school, she was chubby, uncoordinated, and not at all athletic. In P.E. she was always the last one picked for any team or activity. In college she was a math major. (Need we say more?) A few years later, after having two children, her seriously fat-bottomed girl genetics became impossible to ignore.

After an auto accident in her twenties, she started lifting weights to reduce the pain from a hyperextension injury to the ligaments in her lower back. Lifting helped a lot. As a side benefit, it also kept the size of her bottom under control. A shoulder injury from a hard fall onto a concrete train platform in her thirties encouraged her to get more involved in weight lifting. That's when she found out that she was good at it compared to most women.

As a midlife challenge, as she approached 40, she joined a powerlifting team and started training seriously as a powerlifter. She competed and won California state, national, and world championships in powerlifting.

The powerlifting community introduced her to kettlebell training. She was so impressed with the improvements in her fitness that working with kettlebells produced, she became a certified kettlebell instructor and a certified personal trainer so that she could share her knowledge with others.

Over the years Michelle has been able to work with and learn from some of the top weightlifting and kettlebell lifting coaches in the U.S., including powerlifting coaches Joe and Nance Avigliano of the L.A. Lifting Club; Pavel Tsatsouline, who introduced modern Russian kettlebell training to the U.S.; Brett Jones, a top weightlifting and kettlebell coach who specializes in injury prevention and rehab; and Steve Maxwell, an expert coach on applying weightlifting and kettlbell lifting to martial arts, including jiu jitsu, and others.

Now she continues to train and compete in powerlifting and with kettlebells, and she also works with serious trainees to reach their strength and conditioning goals. Note that Michelle doesn't ride a bike for cardio training. Because she doesn't enjoy cardio training, she's opted to do more kettlebell snatching plus some brisk walking rather than riding a bike. She's decided that kettlebell training plus walking provides all the cardio conditioning she wants. Enjoying what you're doing is a key part of maintaining long term training consistency.

When Andy was in elementary school, he swam with the neighborhood pool swim team. He continued to swim in high school and also ran cross country. In college at the University of California—Davis, he got into bicycling and rode everything from criterium races to century (100-mile) rides and double century (200-mile) rides. In all of these sports, he was a middle-of-the-pack athlete.

When he was hit by a car while riding his bike at age 20, he suffered severe injuries, including a broken back, internal injuries, and head and facial trauma. His hospitalization and rehab took more than a year. Afterward, although he was physically able to get back on a bike and ride, he was emotionally unable to continue.

At this point in his life, he turned to his new family and work and turned away from staying physically active and fit. In his mid-thirties, however, he was forced to come to grips with his poor physical shape when his weight topped 200 pounds, 50 pounds more than how much he'd weighed in college. He also suffered from blood clots in his legs and was diagnosed with Lieden Factor V (a blood disorder).

In an effort to regain his former level of fitness, he returned to cycling, though now it was mountain biking. By staying on the trails and off the roads, he was able to overcome his memories of the accident and his emotional hurdles. After a while, he was back to metric century, century, and double century rides on the road. He also began competing in road races and time trials.

Like Michelle, he sought out top coaches to work with and learn from. Over the years, he has been lucky to be able to train under Chris Carmichael (Lance Armstrong's coach), Eddie Borysewicz (1980–84 U.S. Olympic cycling coach), and Davis Phinney and Connie Carpenter (top riders turned coaches). He's also had opportunities to ride with top amateur and pro riders.

In time, he brought his weight back down to its college level and became an aerobic animal.

At the same time, he noted that his strength, which had never been great, was fading as he got older. Michelle's involvement in powerlifting and kettlebell lifting had exposed him to the world of strength training, and now he picked it up and worked hard to improve this aspect of his fitness.

Now he faced the challenge of how to put everything together. Strength training with bicycle riding and kettlebell lifting. Improving all aspects of his strength and conditioning in a practical, doable way.

Andy's main challenge was how not to let strength training adversely affect cardio training, and vice versa, especially given that his recovery ability wasn't highly efficient. After many years of experimentation, he finally found what worked: *focus on one aspect at a time and cut everything else back to maintenance only.* Then rotate the focus over the course of a year. Today, in his fifties, Andy is stronger and in better overall condition than at any earlier time of his life.

There have of course been setbacks. He suffered a broken femur in a bicycle crash and was hospitalized with a ruptured appendix that required emergency surgery. And thanks to that old automobile accident, he still experiences significant back pain on a regular basis due to the injuries he suffered then. But now he doesn't quit. Every time he goes back to strength and conditioning training, he starts at a lower level and pushes forward. Every time, he sees improvement in his performance.

Intensity—the Forgotten Secret of Superior Fitness

The secret to getting fit and staying fit, now and on into the future, is the application of intensity. *You absolutely must exercise intensely.* You may be thinking that eye bulging, white-hot, muscle-searing efforts aren't for you, but please don't stop reading now. Your efforts must be intense, but they needn't be painful. In fact, they shouldn't be painful, because if they are, then you'll start dreading your strength and conditioning training and quit.

We call intensity the forgotten secret of superior fitness because we see so little of it among exercisers nowadays. While a small percentage of serious, fit trainees and athletes get it and exercise intensely, the vast majority who exercise do it without much physical effort or mental focus. Everyone seems terrified of overtraining and/or hurting themselves by doing hard efforts, and so they've eliminated effort entirely from their exercise programs. This is a huge mistake. Without hard, intense effort it is not possible to improve your fitness.

Intensity zones

When we say that you have to exercise intensely, we mean that you need to exceed what your body is comfortable doing, not what it's capable of doing. In other words, need to exceed your comfort zone while staying below your pain zone.

What does this mean? Visualize yourself in the middle of three concentric rings. The ring closest to you is your comfort zone. This level of intensity is easy for you to achieve physically and mentally. It requires little concentration. This zone provides little potential for improvement.

The next ring out is your improvement zone. Your efforts here stretch you physically to beyond what you normally do. They require a significant amount of focused attention. But your efforts in this ring are well within the realm of possibility for you, and you won't hurt yourself. This is the zone you need to be in to make significant improvements. This is the proper intensity.

When we say that you have to exercise intensely, we mean that you need to exceed what your body is comfortable doing, not what it's capable of doing. In other words, need to exceed your comfort zone while staying below your pain zone.

The outer ring is the pain zone. Your efforts here are physically very hard. They're painful. These are the workouts that make you puke and leave you sore for days afterwards. They're mentally difficult because you have to work hard to psych yourself up and develop a high tolerance for discomfort. These workouts are so hard you can't do them consistently, and while you're doing them, you can't really concentrate properly. It's too much for your body and your mind. You don't make any progress here.

Staying in your comfort zone doesn't give your body any reason to adapt and get stronger or have more endurance. It judges what you're doing and says, *No problem, I can handle this.* So there's no reason for your body to add any muscle or make any other changes to itself. But when you stretch and slightly exceed your comfort zone, your body goes, *Uh-oh, I need to make changes to meet these additional demands.* Your body then adapts and makes those changes.

Progressively increasing the intensity in all the exercises you do forces your body to adapt. It will change to meet these new requirements being placed on it. This is the way, and the only way, to get fitter.

For example, if you're able to walk several blocks easily, it's not a challenge to your body when you park further from the store and walk a dozen extra steps. That's why, unless walking even a few steps in difficult for you, those popular programs that use pedometers and encourage people to do eight or ten thousand steps a day don't increase your fitness. We're not saying that walking is bad. Any motion is better than staying completely sedentary. Compared to sitting on the couch (or in front of your computer) all day, walking more will improve your health. What we're saying is that to improve your fitness and to maintain that improvement, you need to make more intense efforts.

If you have any familiarity at all with weightlifting, you've heard of progressive overload. It's a core principle, an alternate way to explain the need for intensity. You lift weights slightly above your comfort level, and then as your body adapts, you increase the weight (i.e. intensity) to keep lifting above your comfort zone.

Progressive overload equals progressive increase of intensity. If you want to get fitter, this is an absolute requirement in all aspects of your training. When lifting weights, you must increase the weight you lift. If you're working on muscular endurance, you must increase the weight used and/or the cadence and/or extend the work time. If you're doing cardio, you must run or bike or swim or cross-country ski or row faster.

What is strenuous, of course, varies depending on your current level of fitness. The fact that your buddy can deadlift 300 pounds doesn't mean that you can. In all aspects of strength and conditioning, you need to find your current levels and work from there.

And always remember to work up slowly from your current levels. Stretch yourself a little every workout, especially during hard workouts, and over time you'll achieve higher and higher levels of strength and conditioning.

But the ultimate bottom line will never change.

You need to perform strenuous efforts
in your strength and conditioning training to improve.

Limits

All that being said, the issue of limits comes to mind. You can overdo the intensity to the point that your body can no longer adapt and breaks down. The breakdown can take many forms, including persistent soreness or illness, an injury, just feeling terrible all the time, or a lack of progress. This issue is so important that we've written an entire chapter on recovery to address it.

As we move into middle age, our bodies' adaptive mechanisms aren't as robust as they were when we were younger. This is why it's vital to balance intensity and recovery, why we have to constantly monitor ourselves. We'll explain how to do this in Chapter 6. You shouldn't exceed your ability to adapt.

Yes, there are limits to what your body can do. Most people don't want to discuss limits, but everyone has them. You have a unique genetic makeup that sets your limits—the maximum size of your muscles, your maximum strength, and your maximum VO2 max. All of these characteristics are normally distributed in any population, which means that most of us are around average, plus or minus one standard deviation.

Only a small number of people inhabit the tails of the standard curve. Only a few people, like Lance Armstrong, have the genetic VO2 max potential to win the Tour de France. Only a few, like Magnus Samuelson, can build muscles large and strong enough to be able to compete in the World's Strongest Man competitions.

A similar small number of people will be below average. Their genetics allow them to develop only minimal strength or VO2 max levels.

Don't let this discourage you. Do let it provide you with some perspective. No one can improve continuously, and only a very few of us can achieve world-class levels of physical prowess. But since almost none of us are anywhere near our genetic potential, we can improve substantially and for many years, even into middle age or older. Eventually, however, we will bump up against what appear to be our personal genetic limits.

When you do this, keep trying to improve. It may be a plateau, not a limit, and even if it is a limit, you'll maintain that level. Our full potentials are unknowable, but they do exist. The idea is to try and reach your full potential. It's a journey that never ends.

We are ourselves examples of varied genetic potential. Andy has always had a light frame. Out of college, he was 5'10" tall and weighed a slender 155 pounds. He has always been more antelope than gorilla. He can ride a bike fast and long, but he has difficulty lifting heavy objects. This reality is a function of his genetics.

Michelle is more of an endomorph with a heavier bone structure and fat-bottomed-girl genetics. She responds well to weight training and is able to lift heavier things than most women her size, but she struggles with aerobic efforts. Her genetic profile is different from Andy's.

A local 26-mile bicycle loop that Andy can easily ride in an hour and a half while chatting with his riding companions would be a seriously difficult effort for Michelle. But she is able to deadlift more than he can, despite being 40 pounds lighter.

> As we move into middle age, our bodies' adaptive mechanisms aren't as robust as they were when we were younger. This is why it's vital to balance intensity and recovery, why we have to constantly monitor ourselves.

Everyone has strengths and weaknesses. Everyone can improve up to their genetic potential. You can work to develop your strengths and overcome your weaknesses by building up what is weak. But try not to compare yourself with others. Developing extraordinary fitness is a very personal effort. Believe the recruiting slogan. Endeavor to "be all that YOU can be."

Almost no one will ever reach their full potential. The time and effort required just aren't humanly available. You will inevitably reach a plateau. Hopefully, it will be a high one. Stay there by maintaining your exercise program at that level.

One final word about genetic limits and potential. Don't fall prey to a common fallacy and confuse correlation with causality. For example, you often hear that if you want to be muscular like a sprinter, you need train like a sprinter. The idea that training like a sprinter will make you muscular like a sprinter is that sprint training makes you muscular. This is false logic. It's just as likely that people with genetics that make them muscular make better sprinters. Being muscular and sprinting are *correlated*, but there is not necessarily a causal link. If you don't have the genetics to develop the muscularity of a sprinter, no amount of sprinting will make you muscular.

Another example that's frequently bandied about is that if you want to be lean and lithe like a dancer, you need to train like a dancer, using movements like those used in Pilates exercises. Again, people are confusing correlation with causality. It's just as likely that genetically lean and lithe people make better dancers. And if you don't have the genetics to be lean and lithe, no amount of "dancer" training will make you that way.

Understanding this fallacy will help you avoid a great amount of frustration. Realize that while you can develop your unique genetic potential to a very high level, you can't change your genetics.

The Need for intensity

We feel that you should always strive to become better. It's the journey, not the destination, that's most important, so when you do hit those inevitable plateaus, keep at it. Keep trying to improve, even if you think that you're at your limits. You might find that what you think your limits are, aren't.

As you strive to improve your strength and conditioning, you will be subject to the many pressures that your life holds for you. Your training must be changed to accommodate these pressures. As a result, your fitness levels will be continually going up and down. You'll need to adapt to your present circumstances. You'll need to reevaluate and adjust your expectations to the current situation.

Life happens. To be successful in staying fit over the long term, you have to accept that your fitness level will move up and down. You need to be realistic and flexible in your training. But you always need intensity.

> We feel that you should always strive to become better. It's the journey, not the destination, that's most important, so when you do hit those inevitable plateaus, keep at it. Keep trying to improve, even if you think that you're at your limits.

The classic study on the effect of intensity on fitness was done by Dr. M. Pollock and associates.[1] This longitudinal study of runners compared master runners (age 45 to 65) over a period of ten years. Two groups were compared. One group kept running recreationally, while the other group kept running competitively. The results were startling. Those in the recreational group on average lost twelve percent of their VO2 max over the ten years. In contrast, among those in the competitive group, the VO2 max measurements hardly changed. On average, they lost about one percent of their VO2 max. The results were clear: only exercising intensely lets you maintain high levels of fitness. Other research confirms the results of this groundbreaking study.

---

[1] Dr. M. Pollock, et al., "Effect of age and training on aerobic capacity and body composition of masters athletes," 1987, *Journal of Applied Physiology* 62(2): 727-278.

To repeat—why were the competitive runners able to maintain their fitness? Intensity made the difference. If you're racing, you train with greater intensity. And you race. Racing provides a level of intensity that can't be replicated in training. Recreational athletes don't experience this intensity, which is why they couldn't maintain their fitness levels.

Other studies done with athletes to determine how best to taper their training before competitions showed the same results. If you decrease exercise volume and/or frequency but keep the intensity, you maintain your fitness. If you maintain the volume and/or frequency but reduce the intensity, your performance is negatively affected.

Intensity is hard, focused effort. In weightlifting, it's the weight used, in bicycling, it's your power output, in kettlebell lifting, it's weight, cadence and time. In every case, it requires concentration on what you're doing. You can't socialize or watch TV or plan your weekend. You need to be completely absorbed in the task.

One of our pet peeves is gyms with TVs where exercisers with pained expressions, in spite of a very noticeable lack of effort, use treadmills or steppers while watching Oprah. And then they wonder why they're not making any progress getting fitter.

> Intensity is hard, focused effort. In weightlifting, it's the weight used, in bicycling, it's your power output, in kettlebell lifting, it's weight, cadence and time. In every case, it requires concentration on what you're doing.

Here's a real-life example. A bicycling buddy of ours on a trip to visit his kids went to a small private gym in the Sacramento area for a few weeks. It's a very upscale gym, filled with rows of gleaming hi-tech machines stationed in front of walls of big-screen TVs. The wealthy clients drive up in their BMWs or Mercedes decked out in the latest trendy and expensive gym wear. They go through the motions, either on their own using the machines or in a class. Step aerobics seemed to be the most popular class. Thirty to fifty minutes, three times a week. These folks are putting in time, but not much effort.

One beautiful summer day, the step aerobics instructor went for a change of pace. She took the class for a brisk, hilly hike over local paths. Half the class, including many long-time members, didn't have the fitness to make it a mile before they had to stop to rest. Most of them decided to head back to the gym. No effort in the class equaled no results in developing greater fitness.

So we ask you, can the average older guy or gal achieve an extraordinary level of overall fitness? Or can only gifted life-long athletes be really fit in middle age and older? The answer: *you most definitely can.* It takes consistent hard effort using good training techniques, but effort that you are capable of.

Woody Allen wrote that ninety percent of success is showing up. With regard to strength and conditioning, that's just partly true. When it comes to fitness, there is one other requirement: *success requires intensity.* Just showing up every week isn't enough. If you want to make progress in achieving superior fitness, you need intense efforts.

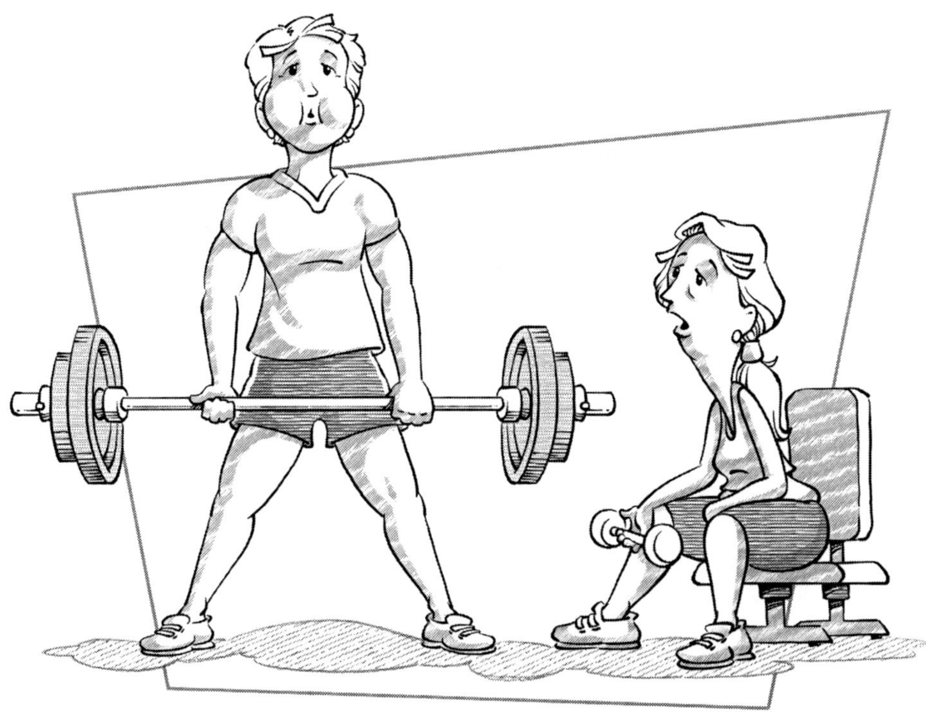

Intensity is the key to fitness.

Andy is a good example. Always just an average athlete, he has stayed active for most of his life and worked intensely. Now this middle-of-the-pack athlete has risen above others of his age. Like everyone else, he hasn't been perfect. In his late twenties and early thirties, he slacked off for many years and didn't get serious about being in excellent physical condition again until his mid-thirties, when his formerly 155-pound body tipped the scales at just over 200 pounds. After that wake up call, it took him several long and painful years to drop the excess weight and regain his former fitness.

But he did it. And if he can do it, odds are that you can too.

2 Strength— The Foundation

Without muscular strength, there is no movement. Strength is our foundation for being able to do what we want to do. Everything we do requires some level of strength, whether it's carrying bags of groceries in from the car, walking, or puttering in the garden.

It's possible for both men and women to get by with minimal levels of strength, especially in modern day America where machines and technology have replaced human effort in almost all areas of our lives. But if you're reading this book, you're obviously not satisfied with just minimal strength. You want to be really strong. You don't want lack of strength to limit your ability to do what you need and want to do.

And that's good, because exceptional fitness requires a base of exceptional strength.

> Strength is our foundation for being able to do what we want to do. Everything we do requires some level of strength.

What is strength?

Most simply defined, strength is your ability to contract your muscles. The harder you can contract your muscles, the stronger you are. For example, two people with the same size bicep muscles pick up a 30-pound dumbbell. One curls the dumbbell easily, while the other struggles and can't do it. The person who curled the dumbbell is stronger. Not because the muscle is larger, but because the muscle is contracting harder.

How does a muscle contract harder? It's a matter of greater neural drive. Neural drive is the brain sending impulses through the nerves to the muscle fibers in a particular muscle. More frequent nerve impulses provide greater stimulus to the muscle fibers, which respond by contracting harder.

Neural drive has three parts. (1) The brain sends the nerve signals to the muscles, signaling them to contract. (2) At the same time, it receives feedback from pressure sensors, including those in the abdomen, the palms of your hands, and the soles of your feet. (3) Based on this feedback, the brains adjusts the nerve signals to the muscles.

Muscles don't normally contract at 100 percent of their potential. This is good, because when muscles do contract that hard, they tear themselves apart as well as tearing from their attachment points on bones. This can be seen in people unfortunate enough to electrocute themselves. The electricity causes their muscles to contract maximally, resulting in severe damage to the muscles, tendons, and ligaments.

Normally, muscles contract at 20 to 25 percent of their potential. Top strength athletes' muscles can contract at up to 40 percent of their potential. That's a huge difference, and the take away for you is that you have a great deal of potential to increase your strength.

Strength as a skill

Strength is primarily a neural phenomenon. It's your brain learning how to contract the muscles of your body harder. This means that strength is a skill. This is so important that it needs to be repeated.

> *Strength is a skill.*
> *It's your brain learning how to contract the muscles of your body harder.*

Why is this concept so important? Because all truly effective methods of increasing strength are based on developing the skill to express strength better.

How do you develop a skill? In a word, *practice*. More specifically, the development of a skill is the result of *frequent and correct practice*. How do you learn to play the clarinet? You find a teacher who shows you how to play it correctly, and then you practice. And the more you practice, the better you get. Someone who practices every day will become a better clarinet player than someone who practices only once a week.

> The development of a skill is the result of *frequent and correct practice*.

In his book *Outliers: The Story of Success*, Malcolm Gladwell observes that successful people are not necessarily more talented, more intelligent, or more ambitious than people who don't succeed. The commonality of success is practice. That is, those who practiced more were more successful. Indeed, Gladwell suggests, it requires at least 10,000 hours of practice in your chosen field to master it and have the possibility of great success. Examples from business, law, music, and athletics seem to bear out this observation.

This also applies to gaining strength. First, you define an exercise that will make you stronger. Next, you learn to perform that exercise correctly. Then you practice the exercise correctly and frequently. As your hours of strength practice accumulate, you get better at contracting your muscles. You get stronger. This is called the "grease the groove" principle. You are creating a groove between your brain, your nerves, your muscles, and your feedback receptors so that they learn to work together smoothly and efficiently. The end result is greater strength.

An idea that is popular nowadays is "muscle confusion." This is the idea that in order to get stronger, you need to confuse your muscles by using lots of different exercises. In our opinion, this is just ridiculous. First of all, muscles can't be confused. They don't have minds. All they do is contract in response to nerve impulses. Second, if you apply this idea, you'll never get strong because by trying to do so many different exercises you won't be able to develop the skill of strength. It's like trying to learn to play several musical instruments at the same time. This is an extraordinarily difficult way to become a proficient musician.

> An idea that is popular nowadays is "muscle confusion." This is the idea that in order to get stronger, you need to confuse your muscles by using lots of different exercises. In our opinion, this is just ridiculous.

Contrast "muscle confusion" with the facts about how really strong men and women like powerlifters train. They practice the three lifts (squat, bench press, and deadlift) consistently for years. That focused, consistent practice enables them to develop terrific strength.

How is strength measured? How strong is strong?

The early 20th century was the heyday of the old-time strongmen. It was a time when men needed to be strong to do the hard physical labor required to live and make a living. A man's strength was measured by how much he could lift off the ground, how much he could put over his head, and how much he could carry. Those were the standards used to evaluate whether or not a man was strong.

Those same standards to measure a man's or a woman's strength hold true today.

What lifts can be used to measure these three standards? We'll leave the standard of how much weight can be carried until Chapter 4. How about the other two?

The world of strength sports can guide us here. There are only a few sports where maximum strength is the most important factor in success. The purest is the misnamed sport of powerlifting (which is more accurately termed *strength lifting*). In powerlifting, the goal is to lift as much weight as possible one time in the three contested lifts—the squat, the bench press, and the deadlift. Contestants develop unequaled pure strength and hoist massive poundages.

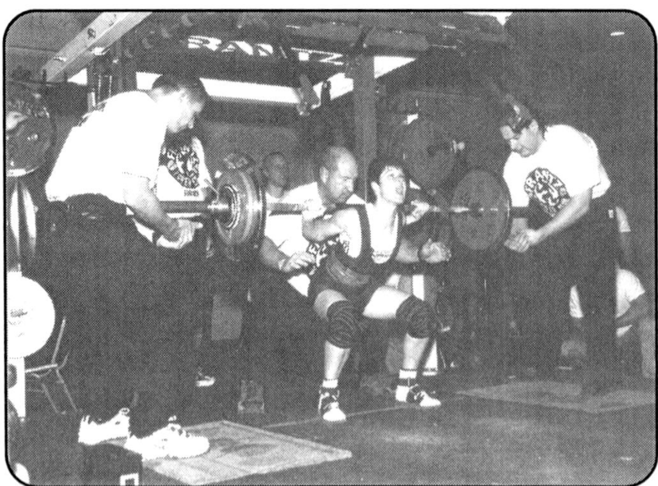

Powerlifting - the squat.

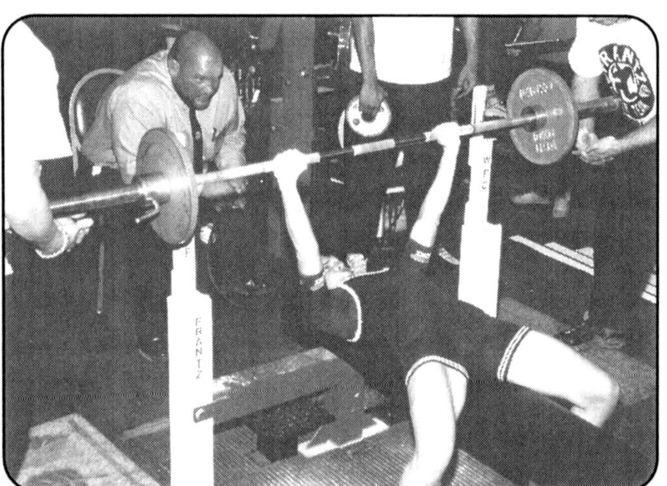

Powerlifting - the bench press.

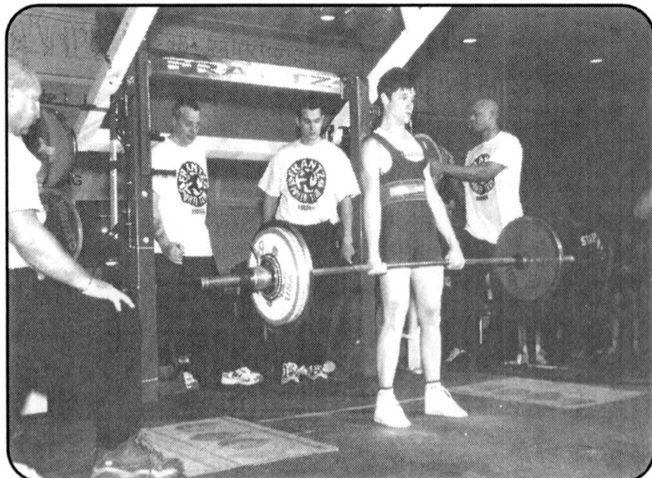

Powerlifting - the deadlift.

In powerlifting circles, the deadlift is considered the most accurate measure of a person's overall bodily strength. This is because the deadlift tests pretty much every muscle in the human body and because it meets the criterion of how much you can lift off the floor. It's the basic lift—you bend down and lift a loaded barbell off the floor.

Let's clarify what we mean by "bend down." Proper deadlift form actually involves squatting down while keeping your back flat, head tilted up with your eyes looking up at a 45 degree angle, and then lifting with your legs, hips and back together. Also, you need to use the proper over/under deadlift grip. This grip prevents the bar from rolling in your hands so that you can lift heavier (your grip won't limit your strength) and more safely (less chance of dropping a lift). It's important for you learn how to do the lift properly, because done improperly by just bending down and yanking the weight up you can injure your back. And back injuries are to be avoided. This is the deadlift paradox—done properly, it really strengthens your back and helps prevent back injuries, but done wrong, it can hurt your back.

Unlike the squat and bench press, where better equipment like suits, wraps, and belts can add a lot to the weight that someone can lift, better equipment has only a minimal effect on performance in the deadlift. Also unlike the squat and bench press, where judging standards have a large impact—was that squat really deep enough? Did the bar really pause on the chest during that bench press?—the deadlift is relatively unaffected by what the judge thinks. It's almost always clear. You either pull the barbell off the floor and lock out, or you don't.

In the world of powerlifting, being able to deadlift 250 percent of your body weight commands respect. For example, competing at a body weight of 52 kilos (114 pounds), Michelle has pulled a 285 pound deadlift, which is 250 percent of her weight. This is a truly exceptional level of strength. If you can match what Michelle can do, you are one really strong man or woman. And it's important to note that this standard applies to both men and women. In overall body strength, women can be just as strong as men in proportion to their body weight.

> To be strong enough for the activities of a normal life, aim for a maximum deadlift of about 125 percent of your body weight. This means you'll be using about 100 percent of your body weight in your usual deadlift training.

But we need a reality check here. Not many people will be able to meet this standard. Our rule of thumb for functional strength is this: To be strong enough for the activities of a normal life, aim for a maximum deadlift of about 125 percent of your body weight. This means you'll be using about 100 percent of your body weight in your usual deadlift training.

If you're an athlete, you need to aim higher. Your maximum deadlift should be at least 150 percent of your body weight. A 150 percent body weight maximum will translate into doing most of your deadlift training using weights around 125 percent of your body weight.

Although the deadlift does a better job at measuring whole body strength than any other lift, it does have one flaw. It doesn't accurately measure upper body strength. This is because in the deadlift the upper body holds and stabilizes while the hips, legs, and back do the actual lifting. For this reason, it's useful to also have a way to accurately measure upper body strength.

Another strength sport that can guide us here is Olympic weightlifting, which contests the snatch and the clean and jerk. This is another sport that's misnamed. This is the sport that should be called powerlifting, since in both lifts the weight must be lifted with speed to be successful. (Remember from high school physics that weight x speed = power.)

In the world of weightlifting, the test of upper body strength is the clean and press. Being able to clean a barbell loaded with a weight equal to your body weight by lifting it from the floor up to your shoulders and then pressing it over your head is the standard for impressive upper body strength for a man. How impressive? It's estimated that less than one in 100 (one

> We believe that the one arm clean and press with a kettlebell or dumbbell is a much better way to test upper body strength than the barbell clean and press.

percent) of men can clean and press their body weight. Some estimates are even lower and in the range of one in 10,000 (0.01 percent). The bottom line is that if you can clean and press your body weight, you are extraordinarily strong.

The clean and press used to be an Olympic lift, but there is a problem with it. When pressing, in order to clear your head with the bar, you need to lean back. This can put dangerous stress on the lower back. That's why we believe that the one arm clean and press with a kettlebell or dumbbell is a much better way to test upper body strength than the barbell clean and press. In the one-arm clean and press, the weight doesn't have to clear your head, so you can stay more upright and thus keep your lower back in a much safer position.

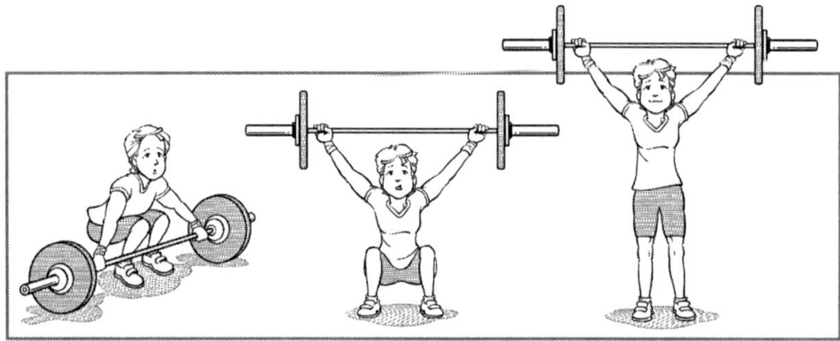

Olympic weightlifting – the snatch.

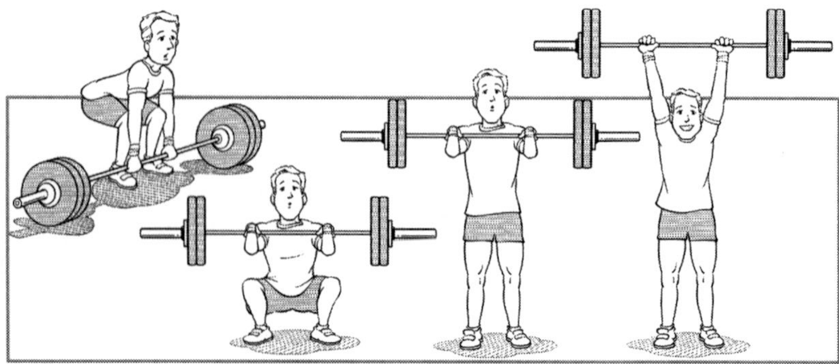

Olympic weightlifting – the clean & jerk.

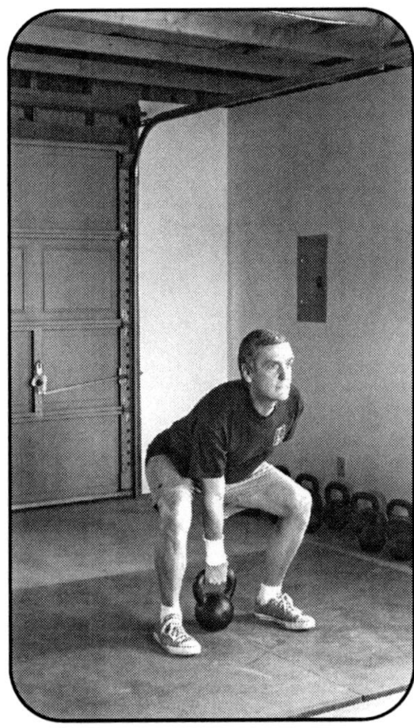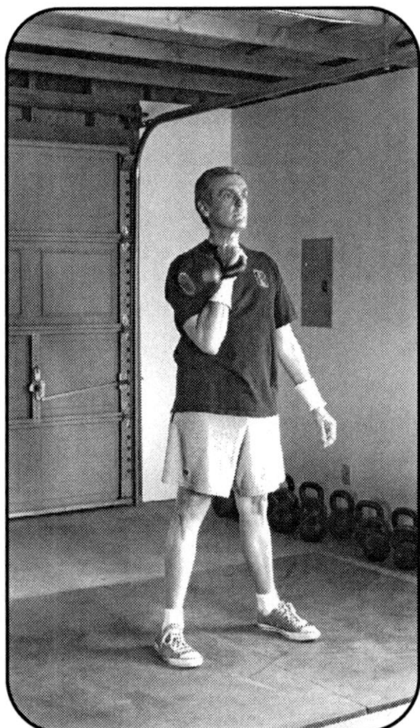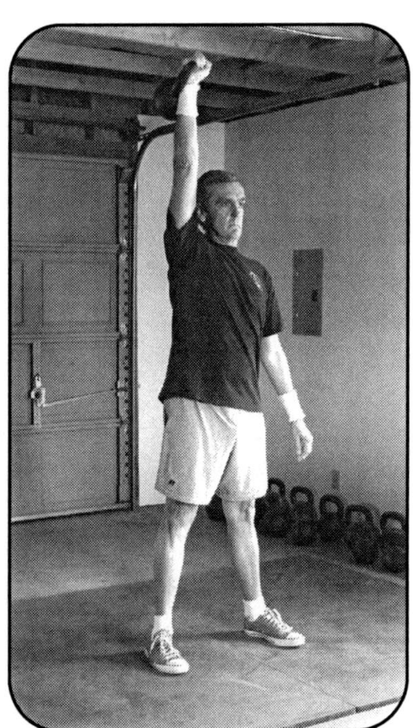

The one-arm kettlebell clean and press.

The standard for a one-arm clean and press for men is 50 percent of body weight. The standard for women is 25 percent of body weight. Women are equal to men in overall body strength, but they don't have as much upper body strength.

And it's time for another reality check. *Not many people will be able to meet this standard either.* To have enough functional strength for daily activities, say, like putting a carry-on bag into the overhead compartment in an airplane, men should aim for one-arm pressing 25 percent of their body weight and women should aim for at least 15 percent.

Again, if you're an athlete, you need to aim higher. Your maximum one-arm clean and press should approach 33 percent for men and 20 percent for women.

Keep in mind that all of these standards are rules of thumb. They're not hard and fast, and other trainers or experts might have different ideas about what the exact standard should be. But the standards we present here do measure strength and provide goals for you to aspire to. In the real world, and especially if you're starting to lift later in life, these standards of strength will be something you'll keep trying to reach, but only a few of you will be able to achieve the highest levels. What to do? Set your goals at either the functional strength level or the athletic level and get to work.

> Don't let the level of your goals discourage you. Whatever level of strength you do reach, it'll be higher if you have targets. If your ultimate goals seem to be out of reach, set intermediate goals to keep yourself motivated.

And don't let the level of your goals discourage you. Whatever level of strength you do reach, it'll be higher if you have targets. If your ultimate goals seem to be out of reach, set intermediate goals to keep yourself motivated. Always remember that it's better to have a target to shoot at than not to have any target at all. You will achieve more.

Many midlife and older trainees have bodies with significant wear and tear on them. We need to take that fact into consideration, too. You need to be aware of your body's limitations and injuries, but even with these kinds of issues, you can get in better shape than you think.

Our real-life examples demonstrate this truth. Andy started lifting seriously in his late thirties. Now he's past 50, and he's still short of reaching the highest levels. At a body weight of 165 pounds, his maximum deadlift is 250 pounds, which is just over 150 percent of his body weight. He can consistently press a 44-pound kettlebell (about 25 percent of his body weight) with both left and right arms.

Here's some background on what has influenced his numbers. His many years of serious bicycling before beginning to lift weights left his upper body relatively weak. Also, the serious accident at age 20 that crushed three of his thoracic vertebrae, which subsequently fused together, resulted in a weak back. Both physical and psychological issues (fear) have limited his strength development. When he was much younger, he was afraid to lift a suitcase, but he has now become much stronger because he has been shooting at those elite strength level targets—the 250 percent of body weight deadlift and the 50 percent of body weight one-arm clean and press By the way, when he started lifting weights, his maximum deadlift was 95 pounds and his maximum one arm press was 18 pounds.

> Many midlife and older trainees have bodies with significant wear and tear on them. We need to take that fact into consideration, too. You can get in better shape than you think.

Michelle's experience was much different. She started lifting weights in her mid-twenties to rehabilitate a back injury from a car accident. In her mid-thirties, she began to focus on upper body weight training to rehabilitate a shoulder injury. That's when she discovered that she was exceptionally strong for a woman her size. Once she started training seriously in her early forties, after a few years she was able to achieve a 285 pound (250 percent of bodyweight) deadlift at a body weight of 114 pounds. And she could press a 26-pound kettlebell (just under 25 percent of bodyweight) with either arm … and not just once. She could do multiple reps with that weight.

An aside—she was also able to work up to a dozen chin-ups. This is an impressive performance, given that less than one percent of women can do even a single chin-up. Again, with a hard target to aim at, she was able to push herself further and achieve more than she ever imagined she could. By the way, her target was to be able to do more chin-ups than one of her powerlifting coaches, who was an exceptionally strong women and successful powerlifting athlete. Her coach was able to do six chin-ups, impressive for a woman, and was amazed when Michelle pumped out twelve solid chin-ups. Also impressed where the guys in the gym who witnessed this contest and who treated her with much more respect afterwards. As a side benefit, this level of upper body strength resulted in her having noticeably large, muscular arms, shoulders, and back that gave her confidence in her male dominated workplace. When she wore a sleeveless blouse or dress, her coworkers could see that she was strong.

Since the days of the old-time strong men, we have measured someone's maximum strength by how much they can lift off the floor and how much they can lift over their head. The deadlift accurately reflects the former, and anyone that can lift two and a half times their body weight in this lift is extraordinarily strong. The one-arm clean and press measures the latter, and any man who hoists one half of his body weight, or any woman who lifts one quarter of her body weight, is extraordinarily strong.

We've presented lower standards that are more realistic for most people. These will still be challenging, but they're attainable with consistent, intense effort.

Now don't rush out right away to find a heavy barbell to test your deadlift maximum lift. Don't run out and buy a heavy kettlebell or dumbbell to test your maximum one-arm clean and press. You'll just hurt yourself. Leave the testing for later, after you've practiced the lifts and developed some strength.

Getting stronger

The first thing you need to do is learn how to perform the Sumo deadlift and the kettlebell one-arm clean and press lifts correctly. This is harder than it seems. The reality is that most of the personal trainers in most gyms in the United States have no idea how to properly do these lifts, much less teach them to someone else.

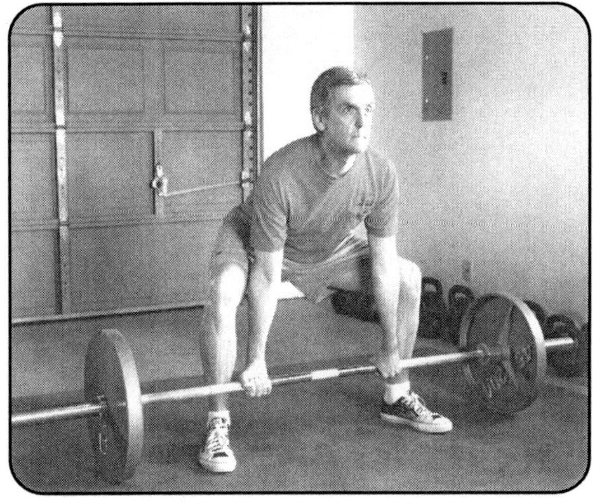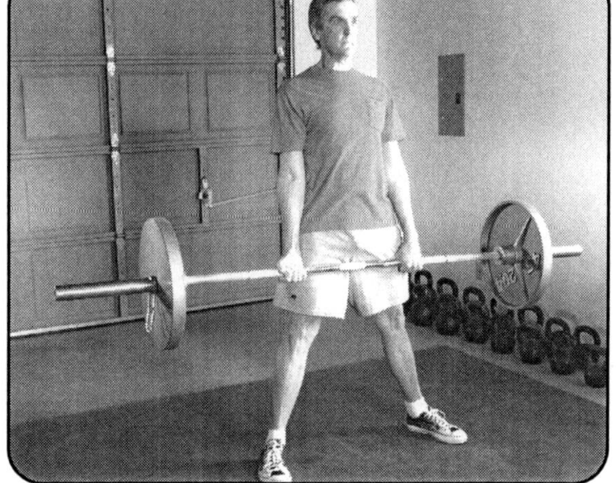

The Sumo deadlift.

You need to find either a certified kettlebell instructor or a powerlifting coach. Russian Kettlebell Challenge (RKC) instructors can be located on the web at www.dragondoor.com, and many cities have a hard core gym where powerlifters train. Yes, we understand that someone who is middle aged and out of shape might be just a bit hesitant to go to a powerlifting gym or to a kettlebell instructor, but trust us — if you go in honestly and openly asking for help to learn how to get stronger, you will be welcomed. Those 5'10", muscular, 300-pound, tattooed guys working out in the gym free weight pit can look intimidating, but most of them are pretty nice.

Ask for help, but don't expect to get it for free. Be willing to pay for a few training sessions so you can learn correct technique. Focus on learning the Sumo deadlift and the kettlebell one-arm clean and press. You'll also want to learn how to perform the kettlebell front squat and the chin-up. (We'll explain why you need to know how to do these additional exercises later.) Ignore helpful suggestions that you should learn other lifts for strength development beyond these four.

> The real secret about why staying focused on only a few exercises can be so effective and efficient in developing strength goes back to the fact that strength is a skill.

There are two ways to deadlift. The conventional deadlift uses a narrow shoulder width stance with the arms *outside* the legs. The Sumo deadlift uses a wide stance with the arms *inside* the legs. Both techniques work, and both are legal in the sport of powerlifting. Why do we suggest the Sumo deadlift? First, it's easier for most people to learn. Second, and more important, it distributes the load more evenly between the legs and the back, thus working the body more evenly and reducing the stress on the back. Another advantage of the Sumo deadlift is that you need less flexibility to get into the proper flat back lifting form than the standard deadlift requires. This is something that less flexible older lifters can appreciate.

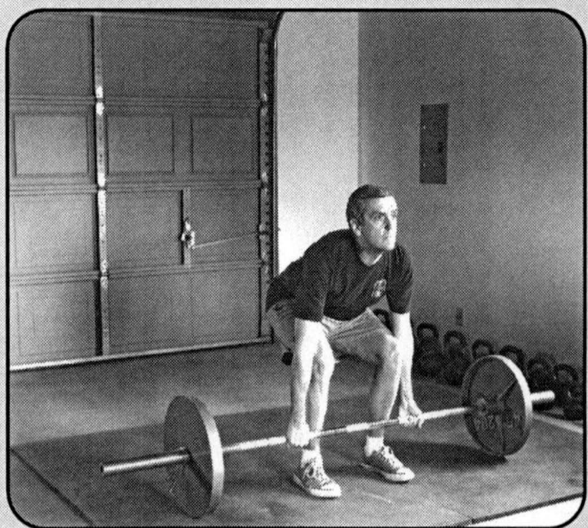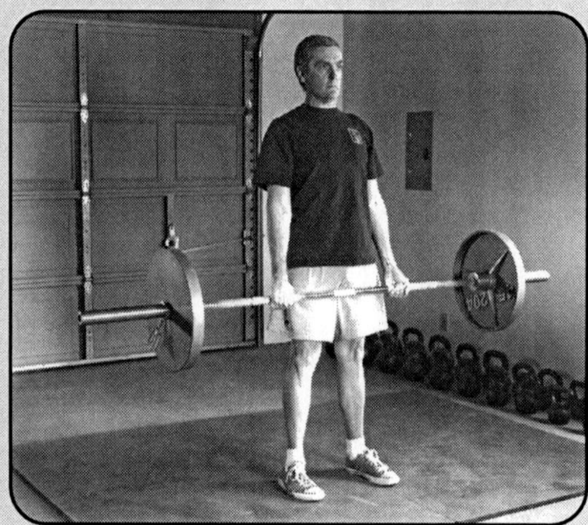

The conventional deadlift – compare it to the Sumo deadlift.

Why such a narrow focus on only a handful of lifts? It's based on the 80/20 principle. You can get 80 percent of results from 20 percent of the effort. The fact is that performing the combination of the Sumo deadlift and the one-arm clean and press works pretty much every muscle in the human body. Worked diligently, these two lifts will let you achieve at least 80 percent (probably much more) of your strength potential.

The guys at the gym will probably tell you that you have to barbell squat or bench press or do lateral raises to get stronger. And, yes, it's true that if you do more, you might get a bit stronger. But these extras will require more time and effort, two things that tend to be in short supply for older trainees. Our advice? *Stay focused.*

And the real secret about why staying focused on only a few exercises can be so effective and efficient in developing strength goes back to the fact that strength is a skill. As you engage in focused practice, you're greasing the groove in your nervous system from your brain through the nerves to your muscles. This develops your ability to express strength.

> Lifting a heavier weight teaches your body to lift heavier. Lifting light weights doesn't do that.

When you have only a few exercises to do, you will be practicing them in almost every single workout. If you fall into the trap of thinking that you need to do many different exercises, you won't be able to do all of them nearly as often. You'll end up doing each exercise maybe once a week, or maybe less, depending on how many exercises you're trying to do.

Think about it. Will you develop more skill practicing an exercise once every week or two, or many times every week? The answer, of course, is the more often you practice, the better—or in this case, the stronger—you'll get. Now, yes, this can get boring. But the goal is maximum effect in minimum time, so you just need to deal with it.

One more issue before we proceed with the specifics of how to get stronger. *Intensity.* In the world of strength, there is only one measure of intensity. It's how much weight you're lifting. The weight you're lifting tells you how hard you're contracting your muscles.

You might think that deadlifting 135 pounds for 10 reps, an effort that wipes you out, is more intense than deadlifting 225 pounds for one rep. It just seems much more intense, right? Wrong. In the world of strength, lifting 225 pounds for singles develops more strength. Remember the definition of strength—it's your ability to contract your muscles harder. Lifting a heavier weight means your muscles are contracting harder.

Lifting a heavier weight teaches your body to lift heavier. Lifting light weights doesn't do that.

So what's heavy and what's light? Generally speaking, anything less than 70 percent of the maximum weight you can lift in a particular exercise is "light." More is "heavy." You need to lift at least 70 percent of your maximum to significantly impact strength.

Both experiments and experience have demonstrated that weights around 80 to 85 percent of your one rep maximum provide the greatest gains in strength over time. This is the level you need to aim for to do most of your strength work at.

Testing yourself

So how do you determine 80 to 85 percent of the maximum weight you can lift without attempting to lift the heaviest weight you can manage? Which is something we definitely recommend against unless you're an experienced lifter who wants to occasionally test yourself or compete. We suggest testing to find the weight that you can confidently lift only five or six times.

Testing can be a pretty informal affair. It can be done once a month or so by replacing a regular strength session with a test session. Load a barbell with a weight and deadlift it five times with good form. Did it feel heavy? If it felt heavy, and you're not confident that you could make a sixth repetition, stop. This is a good estimate of 80 to 85 percent of your maximum. But if can you honestly say that you could've easily lifted it several more times, add some weight and try it again. If you couldn't lift the weight at least five times, subtract some pounds and try again. Do the same thing with the one-arm clean and press using different weight kettlebells or dumbbells. These weights will be your working weights for these two exercises for now.

Guys, you're old enough that by now you should be in control of your ego. Start lighter than you think you should. Gals, you need to be using weights heavier than those 3-pound pink Barbie dumbbells.

Functional Training?

One strength training trend that's currently enjoying considerable popularity is "functional training," which involves lifting weights while balancing on a ball or a wobble board. Because of the instability, light weights are *de rigueur*. This type of training evolved from physical therapy for injured people, and there it may be of some value. For someone just trying to get stronger, however, it's not just useless, but it's also dangerous. It's useless because light weights will not build strength. It's dangerous because lifting weights on an unstable surface creates a good possibility that something will go wrong and the weight will torque your body badly. *Bottom line—DON'T do it.*

Ball training doesn't train "core" muscles any better than training on stable ground does. In fact, a recent study demonstrated that the capacity for maximum core muscle contraction actually decreases when we are exercising on unstable surfaces compared to exercising on solid ground.[2] Toss the balls and train on the ground.

---

[2]*International Journal Sports Physiology Performance*, 4: 97-109, 2009.

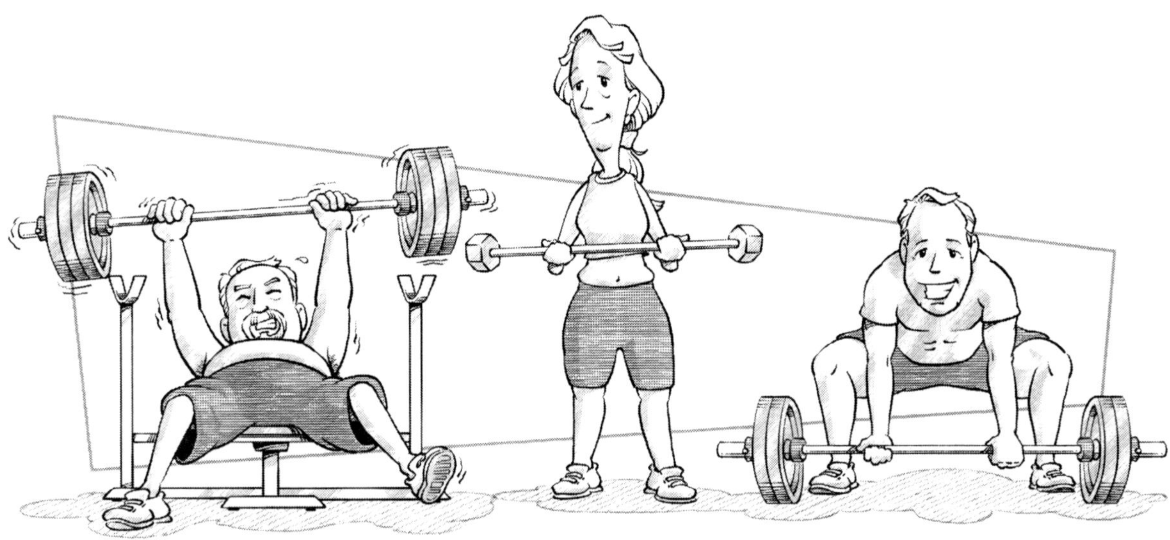

Proper intensity. Not too heavy, not too light, but just right.

As much as we prefer exercising at home, going to a gym for your testing sessions can be a good idea. Gyms will have a wider range of weights for you to use.

The number one rule of testing is to always err on the side of choosing a lighter weight as your working weight. It's never wrong to start with a lighter weight; you will naturally progress to heavier weights as you get stronger. On the other hand, starting with a weight that's too heavy is always a mistake that can lead to injury, burnout, or just lack of progress.

In the real world, this rule comes out modified as follows. Guys, you're old enough that by now you should be in control of your ego. Start lighter than you think you should. Gals, you need to be using weights heavier than those 3-pound pink Barbie dumbbells. Start heavier.

Getting stronger — the details

Now let's turn to the nuts and bolts of how to get stronger. The primary rule of gaining strength is to lift heavy weights lots of times while you're as fresh as possible. In practice, this means lots and lots of low rep sets with long rest periods between.

How low is low rep? For strength purposes, it's one to three reps per set. Younger trainees can go up to five reps per set, but the added reps tend to be problematic for those of us in middle age and beyond. We have trouble recovering from higher rep sets. And from personal experience, we can tell you that sets of five (or more) reps will make you sore. Sets of three (or fewer) will enable you to avoid most muscle soreness. So stick with one to three reps per set when training for strength.

How long are long rest periods? A minimum of three to five minutes. It takes at least that long for the neurotransmitters in your nerves to replenish themselves and be ready for the next set. It also takes that long for the energy substrates in your muscles to replenish. If you can do it, hours between sets is even better. For most of you, this will seem like forever between sets.

With low reps and long rest periods between sets, your strength workouts will not seem very strenuous, but you must remember that when you're developing strength, you're practicing a skill, not working out to the point of exhaustion. It's very difficult to develop strength when you're fatigued. You need to be fresh. You're doing strength training, not conditioning. That's what cardio and muscular endurance training are for. An important corollary is that you must do any cardio or muscular endurance conditioning or sports practice *after* your strength training, never before. You can't do proper strength training when you're tired.

> With low reps and long rest periods between sets, your strength workouts will not seem very strenuous, but you must remember that when you're developing strength, you're practicing a skill, not working out to the point of exhaustion.

How many sets are lots and lots? As many as you can do and still recover from. Experience has shown that for middle age and older trainees, this number of sets is normally between three and fifteen per exercise in a session. This works out to a total daily volume of between three and thirty lifts (reps times sets). Younger trainees can conceivably bump this volume up to as much as 75 lifts in a day, but because of the recovery factor, if you're 40 or older, you're better off keeping the volume much lower than 75.

Which exercises should you use to get stronger? You can't do better than the big pull and press combo of the Sumo deadlift and kettlebell one-arm clean and press.

And which strength training protocol is the most efficient and most effective? Here experience has shown rep ladders are the answer. Rep ladders are both super-reliable in increasing strength and simple to do, and they can be structured to be time-efficient. We won't deny that there are lots of other strength protocols that will work, but we've found that they pale in comparison to rep ladders in terms of getting the most results for the effort expended.

What are rep ladders? You start with set 1 doing one rep. Then in set 2, you do two reps. Then in set 3, you do three reps. For set 4, you drop back to one rep, followed by set 5 with two reps and set 6 with three reps. Continue this 1-2-3 ladder pattern until you complete three to five ladders. When you first start with a particular weight, you should start with three ladders and over time work up to five ladders. If you can't do at least three 1-2-3 ladders confidently and with good form, the weight you've chosen is too heavy. Drop the weight by 3 to 5 percent and try again. And remember the intensity zones: the ladders should stretch you, but not be gut-bustingly difficult.

After working up to five ladders, you should either retest yourself and adjust the weight you're using or go ahead and just add 3 to 5 percent and drop back down to three ladders. Why

3 to 5 percent? Because adding less than 3 percent falls into the realm of being hardly noticeable. It also retards the process of getting stronger. Adding more than 5 percent tends to make the weight too heavy, again retarding your progress and risking injury.

Adjusting the weight precisely by 3 to 5 percent is easy with a barbell and a selection of different weight plates ranging from 1.25 to 25 pounds. It can be harder when you're using kettlebells because they jump up in weight in larger increments. The solution to making smaller increases is to duct tape small 1.25 or 2.5 pound weight plates flat to the bottom of the kettlebell. This works well when increasing the weight when doing kettlebell clean and presses and kettlebell front squats. Just be sure that the plates are taped securely and check often that they are still secure. DO NOT use this trick when doing ballistic kettlebell exercises like the swing, snatch, and long-cycle clean and jerk. These exercises involve high speeds and forces that can loosen even a well taped weight plate. Needless to say, flying weight plates, even small ones, are hazardous.

> Rep ladders are the meat and potatoes of strength training. They should make up almost all of your efforts to gain strength.

When doing rep ladders, always drop down to one rep after the top set. This is not a pyramid 1-2-3-2-1. It's a ladder 1-2-3-1-2-3. With rep ladders, you're doing a mini cycle within the workout which lets you do more total lifts before becoming fatigued. It helps you meet the strength training requirement of doing your reps while as fresh as possible.

To minimize fatigue, the rest periods between sets need to be between 3 to 5 minutes. On the surface this seems impractical. If you were to do five 1-2-3 ladders for two exercises with four minutes rest, your total workout time would be over two hours. You can shorten the overall time by doing the two exercises alternately, starting each set at two minute intervals.

For example, to start perform set 1 of the deadlift, at two minutes do set 1 of the clean and press. At four minutes, go back to the deadlift and do set 2. Alternating like this lets you rest about four minutes between sets of the same exercise and is much more time efficient. Doing it this way lets you complete five 1-2-3 ladders for two exercises in just under an hour.

How many rep ladders should you do? In Chapter 5 we'll explain in detail about "light" (lower-volume) and "heavy" (higher-volume) workouts. For now, just understand that with the rep ladder protocol, three to five 1-2-3 ladders is a heavy workout. Two to three 1-2-3 ladders is a light workout. Of course the lighter ladder workouts will be shorter.

Rep ladders are the meat and potatoes of strength training. They should make up almost all of your efforts to gain strength. But even with a terrifically effective protocol like this, you will get stale and your strength will plateau.

This is absolutely normal. The human body is not a machine. It requires time for adaptation when it's stressed. So smoothly increasing the weights used in a progressive way works until it doesn't.

When it stops working, you have two options. The first is to switch from a strength development focus to a focus on conditioning, either muscular endurance or cardio. Switching is the preferred option, and if this works for you, great. But what if you really want to keep getting stronger? Perhaps you're set on meeting a certain goal you've set for yourself, perhaps you're getting ready for a lifting competition. In this case, you need to change your approach and manipulate your body into further adaptation.

A way to boost your strength quickly

Enter daily singles. Daily singles work not as a long-term training protocol, but for a week or two to break out of a plateau. But daily singles are much harder than they look on paper, so proceed with caution.

What are daily singles? You use the same two exercises you've been using for rep ladders. Or, usually better, focus on only one exercise that has hit a plateau and drop all other strength training. This program is that hard, and it's easy to overdo it. Add 3 to 5 percent to the weight you've been using doing rep ladders, but as the name implies, do only singles. On Monday start with three singles, Tuesday do five singles, Wednesday do seven singles. Continue to add two singles every day until you're doing fifteen singles on Sunday. You must use long rest periods. A minimum of five minutes between singles is good, but it's better to space the singles out during the day. This can be hard to arrange during work hours, but a stay-at-home vacation can be an ideal time for this program.

> After a week of daily singles, take three to five days off before testing your progress and returning to rep ladders.

This program starts pretty easily and quickly becomes very hard. After a week of daily singles, take three to five days off before testing your progress and returning to rep ladders. If you've been stuck at a certain weight, you'll probably be pleasantly surprised at the progress you've made in less than two or maybe three weeks.

Here's an example of how effective daily singles can be. For a long time, Andy was stuck at three chin-ups. He could do five 1-3 rep ladders, but couldn't do four chin-ups when testing for max reps. So he tried daily singles. He dropped all of his other strength training and focused all of his energy on chin-ups. He got a dip belt and hooked on a 10-pound plate (6 percent of his body weight, in retrospect, a bit heavy) and for a week did daily singles with this added weight. He then added another 5-pound plate (15 pounds, total) and did another week of daily singles. As he soon found out, this was much harder than it sounds. But then came the moment of truth. After resting for four days, he tested his max reps on Friday. He did six bodyweight chin-ups. He had doubled his maximum in less than three weeks! That plateau was history.

How to maintain your strength

Rep ladders and daily singles build strength. When you're focused on getting stronger, they're unparalleled. But what about the times you're focused on building muscle and losing fat? Or on improving your cardiovascular conditioning? Or what if your sport's now in season? The fact is that these programs are too intense to use during such times.

If you stop all strength training, you'll lose the fruits of your hard efforts relatively quickly—in as soon as two weeks from when you stop. You need to continue to train for strength. The good news is that while it takes a lot of hard effort to increase your strength, maintaining it is comparatively easy. As long as you maintain intensity, that is, as long as you keep using heavy weights, two strength sessions a week will keep your strength up. As for sets and reps, doing three to five sets of two reps will do the job.

Why two reps? Studies have shown that for almost all people, the second rep of a weightlifting exercise is the strongest. It's the rep on which you are able to exert the most force. The first rep enables your brain to get a feel for how heavy the weight is and send the muscles the right signals on how hard to contract. This is a protective mechanism so you can avoid injuring yourself by matching muscle force with weight. It avoids situations like when you pull hard on a suitcase you thought was heavy, but is really empty causing your to lose your balance and fall. After the second rep, your force production decays due to fatigue until it's below the weight on the bar and you can't complete any more reps. By doing sets of two, therefore, you're focusing on the most effective number to maximize force production and strength development.

> As long as you maintain intensity, that is, as long as you keep using heavy weights, two strength sessions a week will keep your strength up.

This three to five sets of two reps protocol will let you keep the strength you've built so that when you return to strength building, you can continue from where you left off instead of starting over.

Also, doing Sumo deadlifts and one-arm kettlebell clean and presses during strength maintenance can be too much for most people to handle while they're focusing on either muscular endurance or cardio training. This is why you need to learn how to do kettlebell front squats and chin-ups. These are very useful as substitution exercises when doing Sumo deadlifts and/or one-arm kettlebell clean and presses would be too much.

> Common in powerlifting circles, but less so in the general population, are individuals with a "berserker" mentality. These individuals exert the greatest force on the first repetition. Evidently, their nervous systems are less inhibited. They can get psyched up and go balls to the walls right away. Most of us aren't like this.

The chin-up is a fantastic exercise that will both make you stronger and let you know whether or not your body composition is good. It's a complete upper body exercise that works not just your arms and back, but also your shoulders, chest, and abs. In fact, chin-ups work the abs hard and are one of the best ab exercises around. You might not believe that now, but once you start doing a lot of chin-ups, you will come to believe it. The only time either Andy or Michelle has pulled an ab muscle has been doing chin-ups and trying hard for one last rep. In fact, even when Michelle was competing in powerlifting, the only significant injury she ever had was an ab pull from doing chin-ups.

The chin-up is a complete upper body exercise that works not just your arms and back, but also your shoulders, chest, and abs.

Yes, the chin-up is the quintessential most bang-for-the-buck exercise. Worked hard, it will transform your upper body and increase your confidence in your physical abilities.

The difference between chin-ups and pull-ups is that when you're doing chin-ups, the palms of your hands face you, whereas in pull-ups they face away from you.

The difference between chin-ups and pull-ups is that when you're doing chin-ups, the palms of your hands face you, whereas in pull-ups they face away from you.

Chin-ups are a better match for the clean and press with regard to working all the muscles in your upper body. Chin-ups work the biceps (and work them really hard—when was the last time you curled your body weight?), while the clean and press works the triceps. Both, of course, also work the back and chest and shoulders, that is, the entire upper body.

As a practical matter, chin-ups are easier to do than pull-ups. This makes the exercise more accessible to more people and enables better progress.

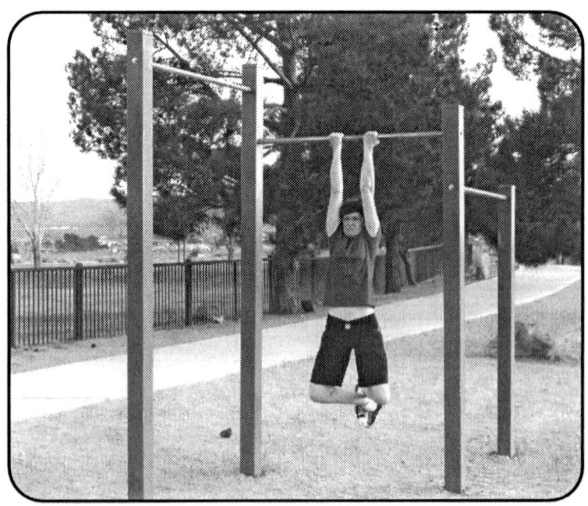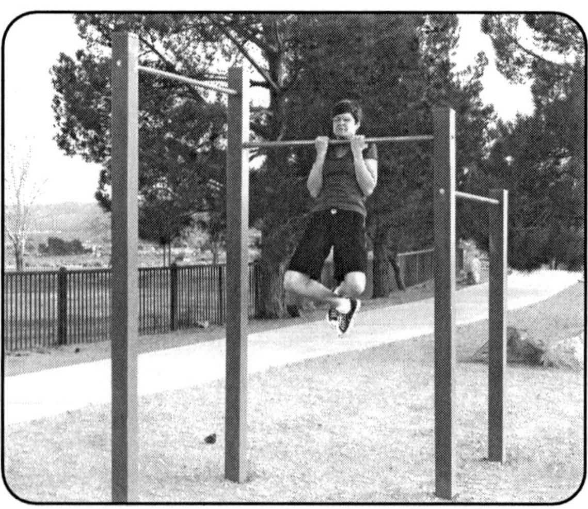

The chin-up.

Also, pull-ups can put the shoulders in an awkward position (especially if you do behind the neck pull-ups or use a wide grip) that can result in injury. Chin-ups with a shoulder-width grip put the shoulders in a strong position, which protects them. This is a good reason to work chin-ups, not pull-ups. An added benefit to using a narrower shoulder-width grip is that your range of motion will be much greater than if you use a wide grip. The greater range of motion will work your back and other upper body muscles more thoroughly.

If you can't do even one chin-up, you can still incorporate this exercise into your strength program. Start with assisted chin-ups. No, you don't ask someone to give you a boost, and, no, you don't need that fancy assisted chin-up machine in the gym. Neither works well in getting you to achieve a true chin-up. Boosting provides too much and inconsistent help, while the machine is a motion so different from an actual chin-up that it won't help. (And don't even think about doing pull-downs on a lat machine.)

> If you can't do even one chin-up, you can still incorporate this exercise into your strength program. Start with assisted chin-ups.

Instead, go to a website like www.jumpstretch.com that sells large rubber bands in various widths and strengths. A half-inch or one-inch band is inexpensive and will give you enough assist so that you can do chin-ups on a bar.

Loop the band around a chin-up bar and put a foot in the other end. Straighten your legs and get in position and the band will give you enough, consistent boost to do chin ups.

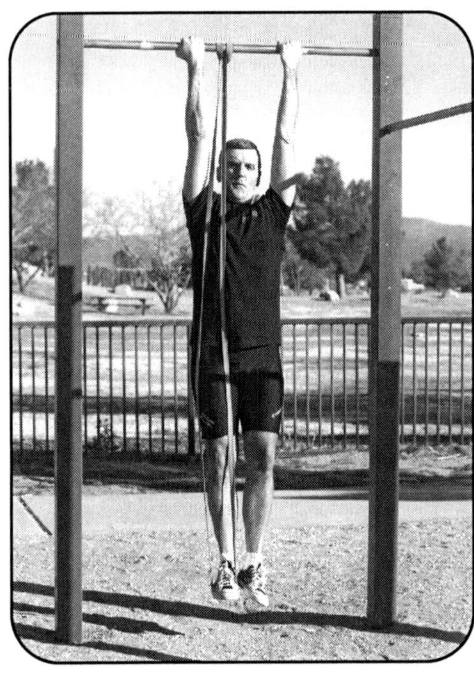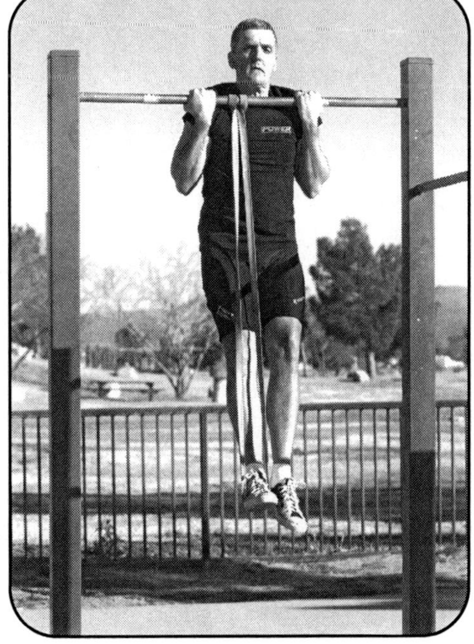

Assisted chin-up with a band.

Of course you'll want to progress to unassisted chin-ups as soon as you can, but in the meantime, an elastic band lets you use the exercise in your strength training right now.

Remember that chin-ups are usually done for repetitions with body weight. They're a strength exercise until you are able to do more than five or six repetitions. Then the chin-up becomes a muscular endurance exercise.

But what we want is to use chins to develop strength. The simple solution is that once you can do more than six chin-ups, you need to add weight. A dip belt with a weight plate or two (totaling three to five percent of your body weight) will reduce the repetitions back down into the strength zone.

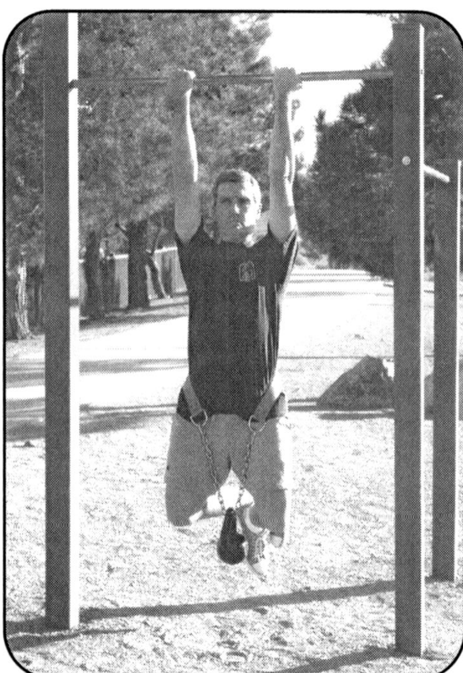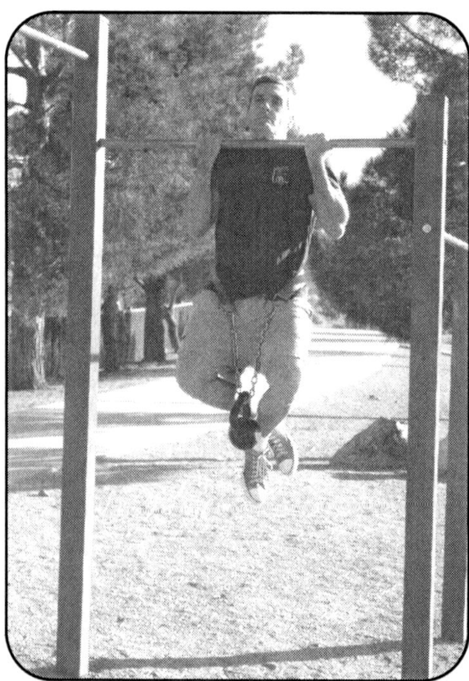

Building strength-chin-up with an 18 pound kettlebell.

The chin-up is a superb strength exercise for your upper body; similarly, kettlebell front squats are an excellent strength exercise for your lower body. Why kettlebell front squats instead of barbell squats or barbell front squats? Because the barbell squat is difficult to master. It's an uncomfortable and potentially dangerous exercise. The heavy weight on your shoulders, the spinal compression, the tendency to round the back forward make it potentially dangerous, and you also need spotters in case you get stuck at the bottom. In addition, there is the tendency to squat down only a little bit instead of going all the way into the hole. (The hole is the bottom of a full squat.)

The barbell front squat addresses these issues because it forces an upright position (if you bend forward, the barbell will fall out of your hands) and forces a full squat because cutting depth (not going all the way to the bottom) is harder than going all the way into the hole. If you

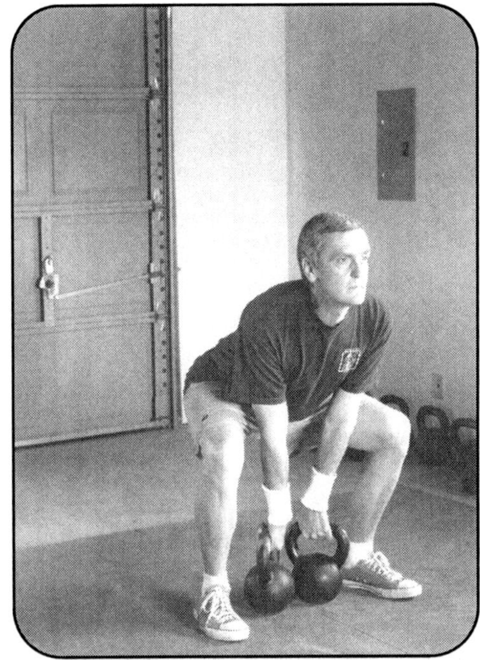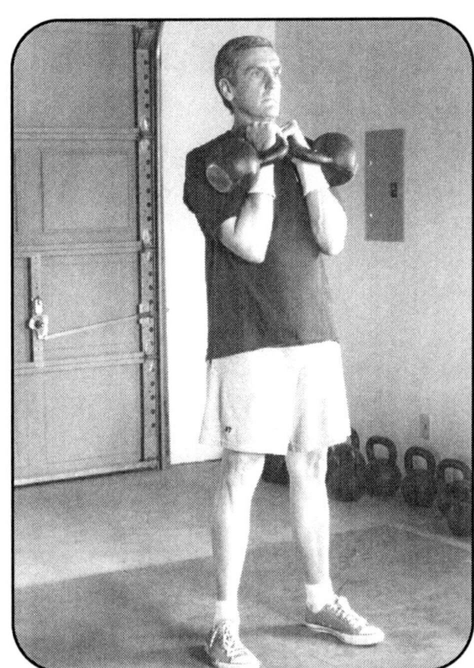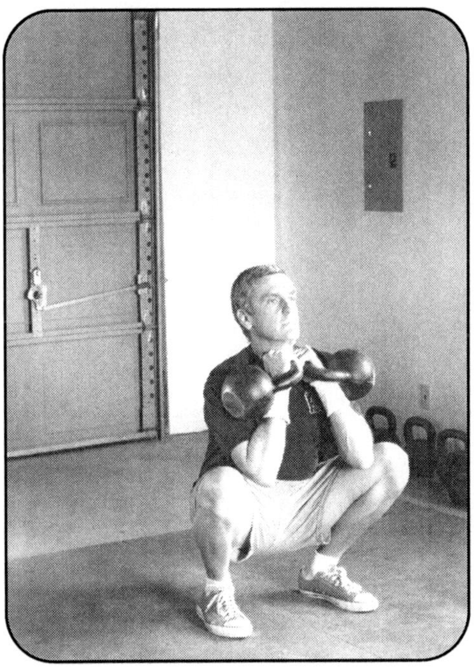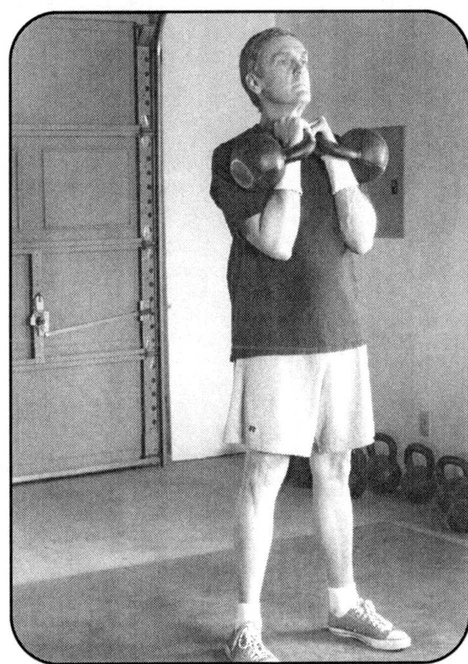

The kettlebell front squat.

get stuck, you don't need spotters. You can dump the weight to the front easily. But barbell front squats are themselves difficult to do because racking the weight on the shoulders is difficult and requires considerable wrist flexibility.

Now the kettlebell front squat has all of the advantages of the barbell front squat plus kettlebells are easy to hold in the rack position on the shoulders. For almost everyone, it's the superior way to squat.

The kettlebell front squat is a superb exercise for developing lower body strength that will meet the needs of most people. However, we want to tell you about what we consider to be the ultimate strength exercise for your lower body. The one-leg squat, commonly called the "pistol." It's a simple exercise – you extend one leg out in front of you, squat down on the other leg until your hamstrings touch your calves, and then come back up. It is a terrifically athletic movement that requires great leg strength, excellent flexibility, and good balance. It can be done with body weight only or, for the very strong, with added weight. For athletes and the very fit, we recommend that they learn and practice this exercise after they've become proficient in the kettlbell front squat. It will take your leg and lower body strength up to the next level. And it's tremendously functional in transferring useful leg strength to any sport or activity that requires it.

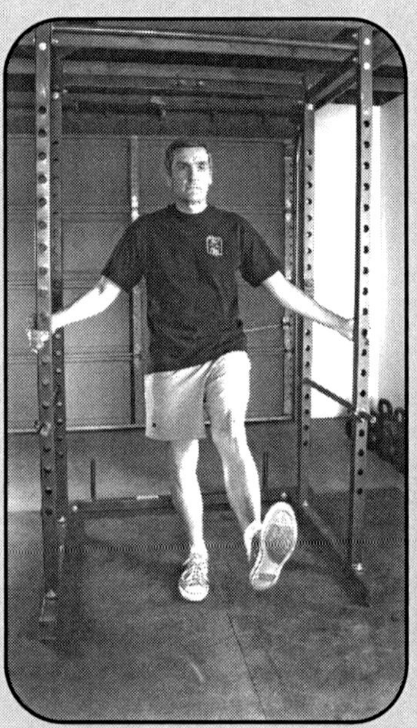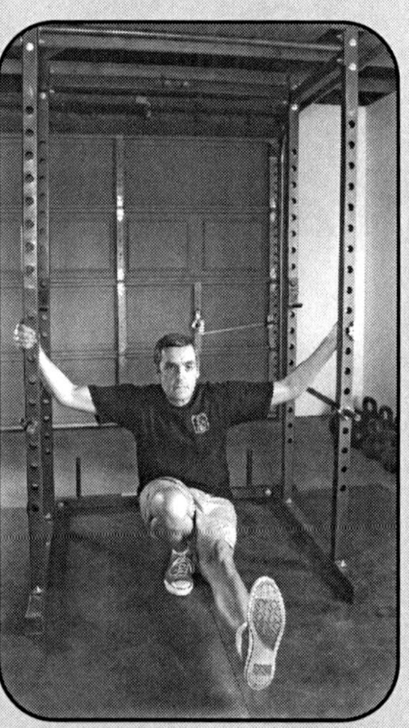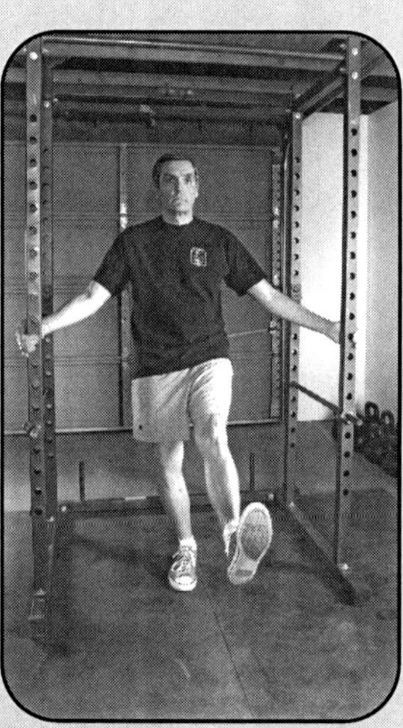

The "pistol"-advanced strength training for your legs.

The chin-up and kettlebell front squat are additional exercises available to use when needed to avoid overstressing certain parts of your body. For example, intense cardio training four times a week on the bicycle will leave your legs very fatigued. Doing Sumo deadlifts or kettlebell front squats with tired legs is not a good idea. Your form will break down and you'll risk injury. Besides, as we've already said many times, building or maintaining strength requires that you and your muscles be fresh. So this is the time to do kettlebell clean and presses along with chin-ups. Your strength training will be centered around your upper body.

Similarly, if you're doing muscular endurance training, your lower back and shoulders will be taking a beating. This is not the time to be doing either Sumo deadlifts or one-arm kettlebell clean and presses. The Sumo deadlifts will overstress your back, and the presses will overstress your shoulders.

This is the time to do chin-ups and kettlebell front squats. These two exercises will provide the stimulus to your body to maintain strength without tearing yourself apart.

This is why you do need to have a couple of exercises besides the Sumo deadlift and kettlebell clean and press in your strength training repertoire. They enable you to continue to do strength training during times when your focus is on other physical attributes.

Incorporate them using three to five sets of two repetitions, doing the exercises alternately. You can continue to use two-minute intervals, but you might consider three-minute intervals instead. Your training won't take much longer, and it'll be easier on your body. And, most importantly, use heavy weights at around 80 to 85 percent of your maximum. Done this way, your muscles and nervous system will stay in the strength groove.

Strength wrap-up

This chapter on strength training has covered a lot of ground. You've learned the basics of strength and three protocols (see the chart, below) that are simple, straightforward, and very effective. You'll get excellent results for the effort you expend.

Summary of the three strength training protocols.

Rep Ladders	2-5 ladders of 1-2-3 reps 2-4 times a week	Build strength long term	Use when working to get stronger
Heavy Singles	3-15 sets of 1 rep daily	Boost strength short term	Use for short periods (1-2 weeks) to boost strength or bust through a plateau or meet a goal
Easy Doubles	3-5 sets of 2 reps twice a week	Maintain strength	Use to keep your strength while working to improve your cardio conditioning or muscular endurance

Let's conclude by reviewing several critical concepts. First, getting stronger requires the application of intensity. In strength training, intensity equals the amount of weight you're lifting. You must lift heavy weights to get stronger. But "heavy" is different for every person. It's 80 to 85 percent of the maximum you can lift.

Second, as you get stronger, your maximum increases. You must progress by adding weight as you get stronger. Test yourself, and as you gain strength, increase your working weights. Or simply add three to five percent when the weight you're currently using becomes easy to lift.

Third, strength training is not for cardio conditioning, nor is it for gaining muscle or losing fat. *It's for getting stronger*. Getting stronger means being able to lift heavier weights. Strength training will have minimal impact on the size of your muscles, but it will have great impact on the hardness, or "tone," of your muscles. Tone is residual muscle tension, and stronger muscles have more of it.

Finally, remember that strength training should not feel like an exhausting workout, because it isn't. It's practice. To get stronger, you need to lift a heavy weight as many times as possible while you're as fresh as possible.

3 Conditioning, Part 1 — Cardiovascular Capacity (VO2 Max) and Aerobic Capacity (Lactate Threshold)

Conditioning is the process of developing your body's aerobic capabilities. Aerobic means "with oxygen," so your aerobic capability is your body's ability to process and use oxygen to do its work. Aerobic conditioning has two aspects—(1) developing a stronger central cardiovascular system (which includes your heart, lungs and circulatory system) and (2) increasing muscular endurance. This chapter is about training your central cardiovascular system. Muscular endurance training is covered in chapter 4.

Developing your central cardiovascular system also has two parts, improving your cardiovascular capacity and your aerobic capacity. Increasing your cardiovascular capacity will increase your ability to go fast or hard. It's the maximum sustained speed you can go powered by your heart, lungs and circulatory system. Increasing your aerobic capacity will increase your endurance, or how long you can go at a percentage of your maximum aerobic capacity.

Cardiovascular and aerobic capacities are physiologically intertwined and both must be developed to reach high levels of central cardiovascular conditioning.

> Cardiovascular and aerobic capacities are physiologically intertwined and both must be developed to reach high levels of central cardiovascular conditioning.

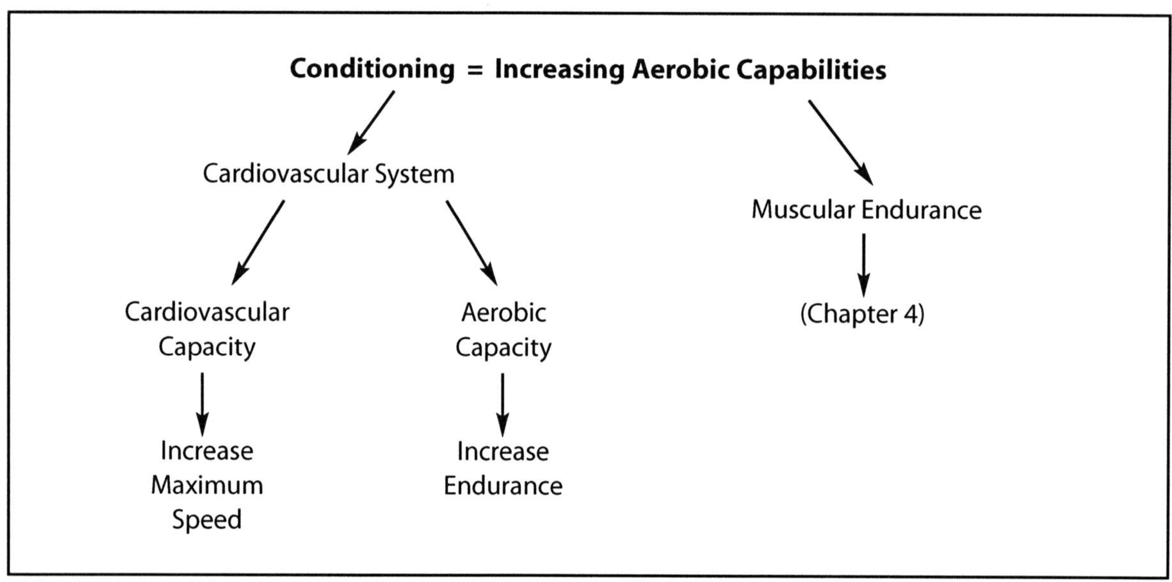

What is cardiovascular capacity?

Also known as VO2 max, this is the maximum amount of oxygen your heart and lungs can take in and distribute throughout your body. It's measured in milliliters of oxygen used per minute per kilogram of body weight. VO2 max is a measure of the capability of your aerobic system. It's your aerobic speed—the maximum speed that your cardiovascular system can sustain. This is the half of your cardiovascular fitness that determines how fast and/or how hard you can move your body powered by your heart and lungs. When you measure your VO2 max, you get a snapshot of what your level is right then.

While VO2 max is trainable up to your genetic potential, there is a strong genetic component to how high you can develop your VO2 max. You'll see this if you measure your VO2 max over time as you're engaging in training to increase it.

You'll notice that at first your VO2 max will increase in a linear fashion, but over time the increase will flatten out. Further increases will then require more training, but you'll eventually reach the point where you can't train anymore because your body can no longer recover from the stress of training. At that point, further increases in your VO2 max are being capped by your genetics.

What is aerobic capacity?

Aerobic capacity, or lactate threshold (LT), is the percentage of VO2 max that you can sustain for a longer period of time. Sixty minutes is the most commonly used time frame. Lactate threshold is a composite measurement incorporating your VO2 max along with muscular metabolic adaptations and movement efficiency (neural skills). It's a measure of the endurance capability of your aerobic system. This is the half of your cardiovascular fitness that determines how long you can continue to move your body powered by your aerobic metabolism. Lactate threshold is much less genetically constrained than VO2 max. Untrained individuals often reach their LT at 70 percent of VO2 max or less, whereas top endurance athletes have LTs of 90-95 percent of VO2 max.

To develop extraordinary cardiovascular fitness, you will need to increase both your VO2 max and your lactate threshold. It's really that simple. All you need to do is to train to improve these two values.

The best way to do cardiovascular conditioning

There are many ways to train your cardiovascular system, including running, bicycling, swimming, rowing, cross country skiing, and rapid kettlebell lifting. This is because your heart and lungs don't care *how* they're stressed, just that they *are* stressed.

But if you're over 40, and even if you're not, you need to seriously consider riding a bike on the road, on the dirt, or on a trainer as your primary mode of cardio training. Why? There are many reasons, but three are of special importance.

> Your heart and lungs don't care *how* they're stressed, just that they *are* stressed.

First, riding a bike is easily accessible to almost everyone. Unlike swimming, rowing, or cross-country skiing, which require special facilities or locations like a pool or lake, or special weather conditions like snow, all you need are a bike and a paved or dirt road. If it's dark or the weather is too nasty to ride outside, you can ride indoors on a trainer. Riding a bike is as accessible as running outside or inside on a treadmill.

Second, riding a bike is superior to running for almost everyone as a way to develop the body's aerobic capabilities. The bicycle is like a time machine for older trainees (especially if you're carrying any extra weight) that takes you back to a time when you were slim and didn't have any nagging injuries to deal with. For younger trainees, the bike lets you get in excellent cardiovascular condition without putting stresses on your body that will become bothersome as you get older.

Pedaling a bike is a smooth motion that's easy on joints and muscles because there is no impact stress. Overall, pedaling has a much lower risk of injury than running. There is, of course, the risk of crashing while riding on the road or trail, but even this risk can be eliminated by using a trainer.

Riding a bicycle puts much less impact stress on your body than running or even just hiking. In fact, pedaling is such a smooth motion that it can relieve soreness brought on by higher-impact activities.

You *can* run to increase your cardio fitness. In fact, using only a stopwatch, you can train precisely to increase your VO2 max and LT. But—and this is a huge *but*—very, very few people can run without injuring themselves over time. This is because to increase your VO2 max and LT you will have to do a lot of fast running. This kind of running puts enormous stresses on your feet, ankles, knees, hips, spine, and pretty much every other joint in your body. There are those few genetically gifted individuals who can run like this without injury, but most people will hurt themselves. This is a good reason why bicycling is a much better exercise than running for increasing cardio fitness.

> For those of you who haven't ridden a bicycle since you were a kid, there will be challenges. In the end you'll be rewarded for the effort you make.

One summer we vacationed in Sedona, Arizona, which is a mecca for outdoor activities. We did a lot of hiking (no running, just hiking). In only a few days, Andy's legs became extremely sore and he needed a lot of Advil to keep going. He also spent time soaking in the pool and the Jacuzzi, but the soreness was so persistent, he almost decided to skip riding any of the mountain bike trails. In the end, however, he couldn't pass on the chance to ride in one of the best mountain biking areas in the country. Because the smooth pedaling action on a bike doesn't create joint stress or muscle damage (and in fact keeps the muscles supple), Andy rode for four hours one day … and except for a sore shoulder that was a result of a crash, the next day he actually felt rejuvenated. The soreness from previous hiking was alleviated.

You can bike a lot and still be fresh and feeling good. Riding on smooth pavement instead of trails makes it even easier on your body. Biking can actually make strength and muscular endurance training easier by relieving the soreness that these types of training tend to create. Your joints and muscles will feel supple and rejuvenated.

A third reason that bicycling is the best way to improve your cardiovascular fitness is that with modern technology, a bike can become a mobile physiology lab with which you can test and monitor your cardiovascular fitness precisely. Using a power meter and a heart rate monitor to get accurate feedback, you can work out at the proper intensities. This enables you to train with pinpoint accuracy and achieve maximum results from every minute of your training.

For those of you who haven't ridden a bicycle since you were a kid, there will be challenges. It will take many hours riding to become really comfortable on the bicycle. A good bike shop can provide you with equipment, like a stable bike with a comfortable seat and low gears, that will make bike riding both easier and more fun. In the end you'll be rewarded for the effort you make.

What you need for your cardio conditioning training

To effectively train your cardiovascular system, you will need sports equipment. Start with this list:

- A good quality bike
- A power meter/heart rate monitor with analysis software
- An indoor trainer
- Accessories, like a helmet, shorts, jersey, and cleated shoes
- Basic repair tools and supplies like spare inner tubes.

Chapter 9 gives more detail on what to look for when you purchase these items. Be aware that high quality equipment may cost several thousand dollars.

You may be feeling some sticker shock.

Take a deep breath. Focus on *value,* not price. The value of being able to effectively and efficiently train your cardiovascular system is huge. Certainly it's much more than any dollar amount. How much is it worth to you to have the energy and ability to do the physical activities you want to do? How much is it worth to you to have a healthy heart, lungs, and circulatory system? The price might seem steep, but the value is truly incalculable.

Measuring your VO2 max

To precisely measure your VO2 max in the lab, you need to be hooked up to equipment that measures your heart rate and the gases expired from your lungs. You then either pedal an exercise bike or run on a treadmill to exhaustion. Your VO2 max is then calculated from the various measurements. This lab-determined VO2 max is the gold standard of measuring aerobic fitness.

But it requires a trip to a physiology lab for testing, which is often hard to arrange and tends to be pretty expensive. Andy has done it several times, but it was a pain. Realistically, most of you aren't likely to go to a lab, especially on a regular basis, which is what is required to track your cardio fitness over time.

The good news is that the trip to the lab isn't necessary at all. It's just not required to structure your cardio training or to track your cardio fitness. While a lab-determined VO2 max value is interesting, it doesn't have much practical application beyond allowing comparisons. Knowing that your VO2 max is, say, 62 lets you compare yourself to other athletes, but it doesn't give you the information you need to train your cardiovascular system efficiently.

The one application of knowing your VO2 max is that it allows comparisons. You can compare yourself to your friends or even Lance Armstrong. Let's do some comparing.

In America, an average healthy but non-athletic man has a VO2 max in the range of 30 to 50. Good endurance athletes, who do well competing in bicycle racing or triathlons typically have a VO2 max from about 50 to above 60. Top endurance athletes at the level of Lance Armstrong have VO2 max values from about 70 to a bit over 80. VO2 max values around 85 appear to be the genetic limit of our species. Lab measurements of top endurance athletes have not found any that have VO2 max values above this.

Interestingly, there are other species that have superior endurance. Thoroughbred racehorses, despite their size, have VO2 max numbers that have been measured at 180. But even they're outpaced by the top dogs of endurance athletes. Alaskan husky sled dogs that can sport a VO2 max of up to 240. Dogs can be amazing endurance athletes, and the casual strolls we take them on don't even begin to challenge their abilities.

> The best way to determine the proper value for you is the most straightforward—test yourself with an eight-minute maximum effort.

So now that you know how you compare, do you feel better or worse? Bottom line? Forget about comparisons. Take where you are and improve yourself.

The really important number you need to know to structure your training and track your cardio fitness is your *bicycling power* (which is measured in watts) at your VO2 max. This is the number you'll use when training to improve your VO2 max. It's also the number you'll track over time to keep tabs on your level of cardio fitness.

Using just a bicycle with a power meter, it's easy to determine your power at VO2 max. Simply ride for eight minutes at maximum effort. Your average power (in watts) for the eight minutes will be a very close estimate of your power at VO2 max. For example, in the spring of 2011 Andy tested himself by riding a maximum effort eight minute time trial. His average power for that effort was 257 watts.

Lance Armstrong's coach, Chris Carmichael, suggests using two eight-minute time trials and taking the higher average power of the two. We believe this approach is problematic, however, because two eight-minute maximum efforts are physically and mentally very hard. You'll tend to avoid testing. Also, almost everyone will hold back a bit during the first effort because they know they'll have to do another one. And then the second effort is compromised by fatigue from the first one. What do we recommend? Just do your best for one effort and use that number as your power at VO2 max.

You can use your power value at VO2 max to structure the intensity of your VO2 max training. While some other coaches and experts suggest basing your VO2 max training intensities on your LT, extrapolating VO2max power values from LT values is fraught with difficulties and inaccuracies. The best way to determine the proper value for you is the most straightforward—test yourself with an eight-minute maximum effort.

This is a maximum effort. It's also long enough that you need to pace yourself, because poor pacing will result in a low estimate of your VO2 max. Compare it to riding in a race. If you start out too hard, you'll fade toward the end. If you start out too easy, it won't be a true maximum effort. A steadily paced effort is optimum for achieving your highest average power output or riding the fastest race that you're capable of riding. This takes some practice, of course, so at first you'll want to test more often until you learn how to pace yourself properly. When you test more often, you'll zero in on your actual power at VO2 max and get a more accurate value.

Pacing is a skill, and as with all skills, it takes some time to develop. Proper pacing is much easier to learn with the help of a power meter. If you start too hard, you'll see your power numbers decline over the eight minutes. Next time, you'll know to start easier. If you can increase your power substantially in the last minute or two of the time trial, you'll know that you started too easy. Next time you'll know to start harder.

It's also important to be using a heart rate monitor when you're testing yourself. Checking your average and maximum heart rates during the eight-minute effort will give you some insight into how your body is responding to your effort. A well paced test will result in a maximum heart rate during the eight-minute time trial of between 90 and 95 percent of your absolute maximum heart rate. Your average heart rate during the test will be much lower, but should approach 85 percent of your maximum.

> Pacing is a skill, and as with all skills, it takes some time to develop. Proper pacing is much easier to learn with the help of a power meter.

So, what is your absolute maximum heart rate? There are three ways to get an estimate.

First, if you're competitive and actively race, especially in high intensity events like bicycle criteriums or shorter running races like 5Ks, your maximum heart rate in a hard race is likely to be pretty close to your absolute maximum heart rate. You'll have to race while wearing a downloadable heart rate monitor to find out what the value is.

Second, testing is another possibility. If you have your VO2 max tested, you can find out what your maximum heart rate is when you reach physical and/or mental exhaustion. Most physicians and physiologists who administer this type of testing tend to discourage people from pushing themselves to utter and complete exhaustion (liability issues). And, frankly, it's hard to come up with the motivation to push yourself that hard in a lab environment. But if you get a maximum heart rate during this type of test, it will give you a ballpark figure for your absolute maximum heart rate.

Third, you can also use one of the many formulas that roughly determine a maximum heart rate. The old *220 minus your age* has been around for a long time, but it tends to overestimate the decline in maximum heart rate in older individuals, especially if they've been continually active. Using an alternate formula, *205 minus one half your age*, is a better choice for active individuals.

If you've been mostly sedentary (be honest!), however, you're probably better off sticking with the 220 minus your age formula. Whichever formula you use, realize that this is a very ballpark figure. But it's better than not having any idea what your absolute maximum is.

As an example, in Andy's case since he's been very active for many decades he could use the 205 minus one half your age formula. This would be 205 minus one half of 53 which equals 178.5 bpm. This turns out to be pretty close to the highest heart rate recorded by his heart rate monitor over the past six months – 182 bpm.

Training to improve your VO2 max

So how do you train to improve your VO2 max? It's simple: perform aerobic exercise at a level intense enough to elicit your VO2 max. Given that VO2 max is defined as your maximum, this will be *very* intense exercise. Exercise right around 100 percent of your VO2 max. Aerobic exercise below 95 percent won't improve your VO2 max. Because of your body's anaerobic pathways, you can exercise harder—over 105 percent of VO2 max. But this level of exercise is too intense. At this higher intensity, it becomes almost impossible to do enough exercise to improve your VO2 max.

How do you structure your VO2 max cardio training? In a word—*intervals*. Periods of hard riding separated by rest periods.

Most trainees find the 95–100 percent range to be optimum. The five percent less intensity may not seem like much, but it makes a huge difference in how physically and mentally taxing your efforts are. Remember our intensity rings. You need to work at an intensity level that stretches your abilities, but doesn't exceed them. For example, if your bicycling power at VO2 max is 250 watts, you need to ride at 235–250 watts (in round numbers). Riding above this range is so stressful, both mentally and physically, that it's hard to do enough to improve your VO2 max. Riding below this range just isn't intense enough for improvement.

Given this information of what your peak power at VO2 max is and that you need to ride a bike at that power, how do you structure your VO2 max cardio training? In a word—*intervals*. Periods of hard riding separated by rest periods.

Many different interval protocols are possible and will work to increase your power at VO2. We prefer to keep it simple. We structure cardio training around only a few different types of intervals.

The first type of interval is a straight VO2 max interval. These are four-minute intervals at 95-100 percent of your VO2 max power with equal rest time (four minutes) at one half of your VO2 max power. A hard workout would be four four-minute intervals, while an easy workout would be half that, or two four-minute intervals.

Riding for four minutes at your VO2 max power is very hard both physically and mentally. An alternative that many find to be easier, but that lets you accumulate the same amount of time at your VO2 max power, are 30:30s. This is thirty seconds at your VO2 max power alternating with thirty seconds at half your VO2 max power for eight minutes. The rest period between these eight minute efforts is half the time (four minutes) and also at one half of your VO2 max power. Each eight-minute interval produces four minutes at VO2 max power.

Because the 30:30 intervals are so short, there's a tendency to go much harder than your VO2 max power. Needless to say, this makes these intervals much more stressful and in the long run less effective. Watch your power meter and aim to hit your VO2 max power as closely as possible.

Using 30:30 intervals, a hard workout would be four eight-minute intervals, while an easy workout would be half that, or two eight-minute intervals. Most of the time, we prefer 30:30s as our VO2 max interval option. It just feels much easier. But we will use the four-minute VO2 max intervals occasionally, if only to build mental toughness. When you know you can go that hard for that long, you start feeling pretty confident.

Determining your lactate threshold (LT) power

Your lactate threshold (LT) power is defined as your maximum sustainable power for one hour. Determining this number by doing a one-hour maximum-effort time trial is really hard, both physically and mentally. For this reason, almost everyone will tend to avoid doing this. That's why we suggest a 20-minute time trial. Twenty minutes is much shorter than an hour and much easier, too, so you can repeat it often enough to track changes in your cardio fitness closely. By reducing your 20-minute maximum power by 5 percent, you will have a very good LT power value that you can use to guide your LT training and evaluate your level of cardio conditioning.

> Your lactate threshold (LT) power is defined as your maximum sustainable power for one hour.

As when you determine your VO2 max power, you use your bicycle with a power meter to determine your power at LT. Ride as hard and as fast as you can for 20 minutes. Ninety-five percent of your average power (in watts) for the 20 minutes will give you a very accurate LT power value. For example, if your average power for a 20 minute maximum effort is 210 watts, then your LT value will be about 200 watts.

As with the eight-minute time trial to determine your VO2 max, when you're doing a 20-minute time trial, pacing is crucial, and keeping a consistent pace will be harder because it's longer. It will no doubt take many attempts before you nail a solid, steady-paced effort. Keep working to improve this valuable skill. This is important because a steady pace is optimum for achieving the highest average power value. A steady pace is also best for riding as fast as you can—it's the most efficient pace for aerobic exercise.

Use your power meter to evaluate every 20-minute time trial test you do to determine whether you started too fast and faded at the end or started too easy and were able to pick up the pace significantly at the end. Over time, you'll learn to pace yourself, which will let you very accurately track both your VO2 max and LT values. In the beginning, use the numbers that the test results give you, but realize that they may be off a bit until you get the pacing down. However, even these numbers will give you a more accurate evaluation of your cardio fitness than estimates or percentages will.

Training to improve your lactate threshold

Once you've determined your power at LT, what intensity should you train at? Improving your LT requires you to perform aerobic exercise at your LT power level. Compared to improving your VO2 max, improving your LT is easier because the exercise is less intense, but harder because it needs to be done for much longer time intervals. Your LT power is a percentage of your VO2 max power. It can range from 70 percent or less of VO2 max in people with poor cardio fitness to 90-95 percent of VO2 max in top endurance athletes. Improving your LT means that you can sustain a higher percentage of your VO2 max for an extended period of time. The purpose of LT training is to increase the percentage of VO2 max you can sustain. This is what increases your endurance capabilities.

Because your LT power is a sub-maximal effort, you can train at 100 percent of your LT power without great difficulty. Training at this level will improve your LT. Doing intervals at LT power is hard, but it's not a maximal effort like doing intervals at your VO2 max power.

Straight LT intervals are eight-minute intervals at 100 percent of your LT power with half time (four-minute) rest periods at one half of your LT interval power. A hard workout would be four eight-minute intervals. An easy workout would be two eight-minute intervals.

As with VO2 max training, training slightly below your LT is easier and also effective in boosting your LT. Riding a bike at 90 percent of your LT power is effective in increasing LT at a lower physiological and psychological cost than riding at 100 percent of your LT power. This means that you'll be able to do more training at this 90 percent pace, which can create larger improvements in LT.

> Improving your LT means that you can sustain a higher percentage of your VO2 max for an extended period of time. The purpose of LT training is to increase the percentage of VO2 max you can sustain. This is what increases your endurance capabilities.

We call 90 percent of your LT power your *tempo pace*. This is a fast endurance pace that you can sustain for long periods of time. It's the pace you use, for example, for long climbs of 20 minutes to three hours or more. Where we live, along the eastern Sierra Mountains in California, we can enjoy riding up mountain roads ranging from a mere three miles to over 25 miles. Your tempo pace is also the pace you use when riding your bike into a strong headwind. (Headwinds of 20 to 25 mph are

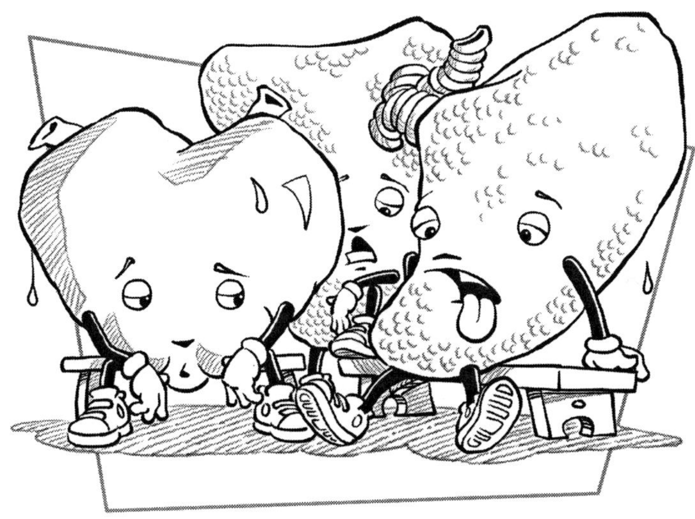

Man, those intervals are tough!

common here in the high desert.) And your tempo pace is the pace that'll let you hang on when you're participating in strong group rides or riding a fast century. Riding at your tempo pace will boost your endurance and LT power, but you need to spend lots of time riding at that pace. When you're training, you'll need to accumulate at least 20 minutes at your tempo pace in a single workout. And an hour or more isn't too much.

To do tempo intervals, which are LT intervals, in a more structured fashion you can ride one to three 20-minute tempo level intervals with 10-minute rest intervals during a workout.

An alternate way to determine your power at VO2 max and LT

Thanks to modern technology, if you race or ride in competitive groups or events, you no longer need to do any testing to pinpoint your power at VO2 max and LT. You can use a power meter to collect your power data, and new software that analyzes this data in detail is now available and becoming widespread. For any race or ride, this software can identify your peak eight-minute power and your peak 20-minute power. It can identify the peak power for any time interval, of course, but these are the two intervals that let us identify our power at VO2 max and LT. Almost every power meter now comes with analysis software that identifies peak powers, and there is also third party software available that can do the calculations using data from many different power meters.

> Your peak eight-minute power is your power at VO2 max. Ninety-five percent of your peak 20-minute power is your power at LT.

Power Meter Software Generated Peak Power Curve

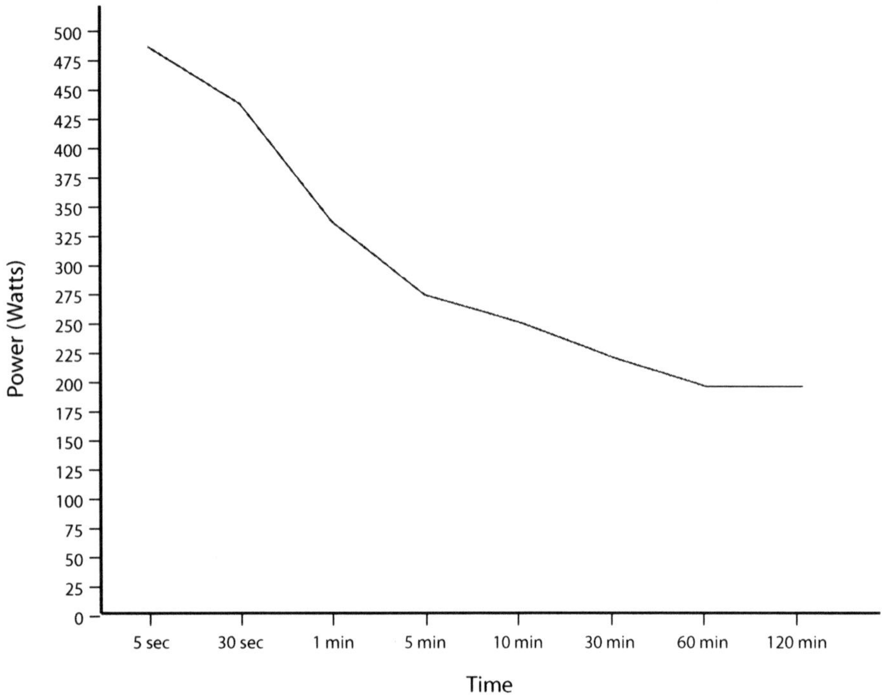

Your peak eight-minute power is your power at VO2 max. Ninety-five percent of your peak 20-minute power is your power at LT. We use 20 minutes because 60-minute maximum efforts are rare, whereas maximum 20-minute efforts are much more common. More data points will provide you with a more accurate value. By reducing the 20-minute peak power by five percent, we get a number that reflects true 60-minute peak power.

Best of all, this software keeps track of these peak powers for every recorded race or ride, so you can track your peak powers over time and see if they're increasing (great—your training is working) staying the same (maybe you're in maintenance mode in your cardio training, so it's OK), or decreasing (something's wrong, but you know that right away and can decide what action to take).

This combination of power meter data and powerful analysis software is completely changing cardio training. You can now track changes in your cardio fitness in detail and in real time. It's more accurate than using percentages to identify your power at VO2 max and LT. It's hard to overstate how revolutionary this is! And best of all, it's available to you now at a cost way below its value.

Bottom line—you must take advantage of this technology. It truly is revolutionary and will exponentially improve your cardio fitness by completely changing the way you train.

> This combination of power meter data and powerful analysis software is completely changing cardio training.

Training your VO2 max and LT at the same time

You can also include intervals that train both your VO2 max and LT at the same time during your bicycle rides. This is called a combination (or combo) interval. Combo intervals are a mixture of time at LT and VO2 max. They are eight-minute intervals starting with three minutes at your LT pace, then one minute at your VO2 max pace, then another three minutes at your LT pace, and finishing with one more minute at your VO2 max pace. The rest periods are half time (four minutes) at one half the easier (LT) pace power. A hard workout would be four eight-minute intervals. An easy workout would be half that, or two eight-minute intervals. Alternating varied intensities in the same interval also lets you get used to changes of pace and is very useful if you race or participate in group rides in which the pace is constantly changing.

Combo intervals also provide a change of pace from straight LT or VO2 intervals. And they can be used as an easier way to do VO2 max training.

> Combo intervals also provide a change of pace from straight LT or VO2 max intervals. And they can be used as an easier way to do VO2 max training.

Structuring your cardio training

So far we've outlined basic intervals that you can use to improve your VO2 max and your LT.

We chose the four-minute, eight-minute and 20-minute interval times because they are mid-range in what studies have shown to be effective and what coaches suggest to their athletes. Other interval times would undoubtedly also work, but we prefer to keep it simple by sticking to one number. The number of intervals in a workout is also mid-range of suggested total work time in a workout. The rest periods and power during the rest periods are also what have been used and shown to be effective.

So now how do you structure your cardio training? The basic principle is that every week needs to include some intense cardio training. This means doing intervals. Doing hard efforts separated by rest periods. You need to do intervals like those we've described above every week. Yes, you need to do the work. Consistently doing intense cardio training every week is the tough part.

How many intervals do you need to do? This will vary with each individual and whether you're trying to improve your cardio conditioning or just maintain your current level. As a rule of thumb, we suggest 30 to 90 minutes of intervals (some combination of VO2 max and LT) per week as a range that works for most people. The lower end works for less experienced, less fit riders and/or when maintenance is the goal, and the higher end is for experienced, fit riders and/or when improvement is the goal.

However, with the advent of power meters we can now be much more precise as to how many intervals are required to achieve a solid week of training appropriate to your level of fitness and your cardio training objective. A solid week of cardio training is one in which you accumulate a sufficient amount of time at your VO2 max and your LT. But how much time is sufficient? It's the amount of time that results in improvements in both your power at VO2 max and LT without overstressing your body to the point that you can't recover from the training.

Finding this balance between enough for improvement, but not too much to recover from used to be a trial and error proposition. All we had to go by was rules of thumb. But not anymore. Thanks to the advanced power meter analysis software, we told you about earlier, a "solid" week of training can be quantified into a single number.

That number is the training stress score (TSS), which quantifies the intensity and volume of the ride and the stress that the combination puts on your body. It does this by incorporating your power at LT into the analysis formula. It begins by defining riding at your power at LT for one hour as 100 TSS points. This means that if a ride scores 50 TSS points, it was half as strenuous as riding at your LT power for one hour. The ride could be longer than an hour, but at a lower intensity, or it could be shorter at a higher intensity. Whatever the combination of time and intensity, the physiological stress on your body was half as much as a 100 TSS effort.

The TSS score was developed by Hunter Allen and Andrew Coggan, and the equation is given in their book, *Training and Racing with a Power Meter*. The equation is complex and incorporates time, normalized power, an intensity factor, and your functional threshold power. If you want the details, you can look them up in that book. The good news is that you only need to understand the concept and appreciate its power, because the actual calculation is done by the power meter analysis software. Many of the analysis programs include TSS score calculations. This is a vital feature to look for when selecting a power meter and power meter analysis software.

> Since the TSS is personalized to your cardio fitness, we can precisely determine what constitutes a solid week of training.

Since the TSS is personalized to your cardio fitness, we can precisely determine what constitutes a solid week of training. During a cardio fitness improvement phase (three or four or more rides per week), a solid week of training is accumulating 350 to 700 TSS points. During times when your goal is to maintain your cardio fitness (two or three rides per week), a solid week would be about half that (175 to 350 TSS points).

These TSS point levels are what experienced endurance athletes with many years of training in sports like bicycling or triathlon achieve in their training when working for improvement or maintenance. If you're new to cardio training or have less experience, you need to set point goals that are a fraction of these numbers. A good place to consider starting would be half. Or you could start at whatever TSS value you're currently achieving. Then, to see continued improvement, work up as required.

You need to do enough intervals in a week to achieve your goal TSS points. This may be 24 minutes of VO2 max intervals plus 16 minutes of LT intervals, or eight minutes of VO2 max intervals plus 60 minutes of tempo intervals. Or it might be 40 minutes of combo intervals. As long as you're doing both VO2 max and LT intervals during a week, it can be any combination that meets your TSS point goal.

Setting and achieving a goal of TSS points every week will give you a precise measurement of what a solid week of training is for you. Increasing your goal points will drive you to achieving continued improvement in your VO2 max and LT power levels.

The skill of pedaling

Pedaling a bicycle is a skill that you need to develop. The ability to pedal smoothly over a wide range of cadences is needed to generate the high power levels that are needed to increase your VO2 max and LT.

Inexperienced bicyclists tend to pedal in a choppy manner at low cadences around 60 rpm. To become a better cyclist and be able to generate the powers necessary to improve your cardio fitness, you need to learn how to pedal more smoothly and faster.

Pedaling smoothly means that you're coordinating all of the muscles in your legs including your quadriceps, hamstrings, glutes and calves to apply smooth power to the pedals. Pedaling with your heel down you start to push down with your quadriceps as the pedal comes over the twelve o'clock position, then as it reaches the six o'clock position you scrape the pedal back using your hamstrings and glutes. After scraping, you relax all of the muscles in that leg so that you're not working against the power stroke of the opposite leg. You can see that this is a complicated coordinated motion that will take time to learn. You need to work on this skill because if you just mash down alternately with each leg, like many inexperienced cyclist do, your pedaling will be inefficient so that you will not be able to generate higher levels of power and you will fatigue much, much faster.

At low power levels, the most efficient cadence is around 75 rpm. This is what you'll use when you ride easy at 90 percent or less of your LT power. At medium power levels, the most efficient cadence is around 85 rpm. This would be when riding at your LT power level. At high power levels, the most efficient cadence is around 95 rpm. This is the cadence you use when riding at VO2 max power levels or higher.

How will you know how fast you're pedaling? Again, technology comes to the rescue. Your power meter will measure how fast you're pedaling and display your rpms. When you can see that number, you can develop the ability to pedal at a wide range of cadences.

So why is being able to pedal faster necessary to generate high power levels? When you're pedaling, you can generate more power by either pushing harder on the pedals or by pedaling faster. If you try to generate more power by pushing down harder on the pedals, it puts a lot of stress on your leg muscles, which requires great strength and causes them to fatigue relatively quickly. But if you generate more power by pedaling faster, the force required on each pedal stroke is less, so you have less muscular fatigue. Pedaling faster does put more stress on your central cardiovascular system (heart and lungs), but it's much more resistant to fatigue than your skeletal muscles are. By using your central cardiovascular system instead of your leg muscles, you can generate high power levels much more easily and for much longer periods of time.

The bottom line is that you need to practice pedaling faster so that you become comfortable and smooth at a wide range of cadences from 70 to 100 rpm. Every time you ride, practice pedaling smoothly at higher rpms and remember that it will take about 10,000 hours of pedaling to really master this skill and that in the meantime every hour of practice will make you better and move you towards reaching this goal.

A valuable technique taught by top bicycling coaches that can reduce leg muscle fatigue even more than just pedaling faster is five-count pedaling. This technique enables you to pedal harder with less fatigue. You count your pedal strokes 1-2-3-4-5, 1-2-3-4-5, etc., every time you push down on a pedal. On 1-2-3, you push hard, then on 4 and 5 you ease up. This technique gives your leg muscles a little rest between hard efforts, and that means your legs can generate more power for longer times than if you just pedal hard all the time. More power, of course, means more speed.

The science behind this technique is straightforward. When your muscles contract, the blood vessels in them are constricted, which prevents your blood from providing nutrients (oxygen, glucose, fats) and removing waste products (carbon dioxide, lactic acid) from the muscles. This results in the muscles becoming more quickly fatigued. When you let the muscles relax regularly, the blood vessels open up, allowing the blood to provide the muscle cells with needed nutrients and remove the waste products. This enables your muscles to work harder longer.

When you master the five-count pedaling technique, you will immediately be riding stronger with more power and less fatigue.

Cardio training weekly schedule

Effective cardio training requires that you train at least two times a week. As long as both days include enough hard efforts (intervals) to reach your goal TSS score, training twice a week will let you maintain your current cardio conditioning. Training three to four times a week is the sweet spot where you can increase your cardio fitness substantially for the time and effort expended. Doing cardio training five or more times a week will bring further improvement in your cardio fitness, but at a slower rate. For most people, riding three or four times a week will bring about the 80 percent of results for 20 percent of the effort as far as improved cardio conditioning is concerned.

Here are the components of a weekly schedule:

- Hard-interval day – high volume of VO2/LT/combo intervals
- Easy-interval day – low volume of VO2/LT/combo intervals
- Endurance day – endurance ride, with 20 to 60 minutes at tempo pace
- Fun day – social group or family ride, recreational event, century, hard group ride, race, anything nonstructured.

Here's how to build a weekly schedule:

- If you plan to ride twice in the week, include one hard interval day and one easy interval day.
- If you plan to ride three days in the week, include one hard interval day, one easy interval day, and one endurance day.
- If you plan to ride four days in the week, include one hard interval day, one easy interval day, one endurance day, and one fun day.
- If you plan to ride five to seven days in the week, include one hard interval day, one easy interval day, one endurance day, and two to four fun days.

Fun days may be unstructured, but they're an important part of weekly cardio training. Social group rides and family rides are very easy and can help you recover from the interval and endurance days. Racing and hard group rides are ways to stretch your VO2 max training. Long rides stretch your LT endurance training.

For complete cardio training, you need to do both VO2 max efforts and LT efforts. You have a lot of flexibility as to how you distribute these efforts throughout a week.

Just make sure that you do both VO2 max and LT efforts.

By the way, you probably won't be tempted to do only VO2 max efforts because they're so hard, but it's easy to get lazy and do only the easier LT and tempo efforts. If you do this, your endurance ability will improve, but your VO2 max won't. Always remember that the gold standard measure of your cardio fitness is your VO2 max. Getting this number up and keeping it there needs to be a priority.

What kind of time commitment are we talking about here? It can vary widely depending on how many days a week you ride and what kinds of rides you do. On the long end, you could ride twice during the week for 1.5 hours and then two to three hours both Saturday and Sunday, which might total eight hours for the week. Or mid-range, you could do two shorter one-hour rides during the week and a longer two-hour ride on Saturday, which might total four hours. On the short end, you could ride once during the week for 0.5 hours and once on Saturday for 1.5 hours for two hours, total.

The bottom line is that you need to structure your week to accomplish your goals with the time that you have available. Set a TSS score goal and structure your weekly rides and intervals to reach that goal. If you have limited time, you can reach your goal by working shorter but harder. If you have more time, you can reach it by working longer and easier. Or if you're really pressed for time, you may have to dial back your TSS score objective with the realization that your cardio fitness will suffer.

> Always remember that the gold standard measure of your cardio fitness is your VO2 max. Getting this number up and keeping it there needs to be a priority.

Sample cardio training weeks

Building cardio fitness.

When you're riding your bike four times a week and working to improve your cardio fitness, you could do one hard interval ride of at least one hour (interval time plus warm up and cool down) with four eight-minute 30:30 VO2 max intervals, one easy interval ride of at least 40 minutes (interval time plus warm up and cool down) with two eight-minute LT/VO2 max combo intervals, one endurance ride of at least 40 minutes (interval time plus warm up and cool down) with 20 minutes at tempo pace, and a social or group ride of any comfortable length. If completed at accurate power levels for you, that would be a solid week of cardio efforts that will improve your cardio conditioning. Again, many other combinations are possible and will work as long as you're putting in both VO2 max and LT efforts.

Building Cardio Fitness – riding 4 days a week.

__Monday__	__Tuesday__	__Wednesday__	__Thursday__	__Friday__	__Saturday__	__Sunday__
Rest Day	Weights & Kettlebells	Bike 60 min with 2x8 min combo intervals	Bike 60 min with 20 min tempo interval	Weights & Kettlebells	Bike 90 min with 4x8 min 30:30 intervals	Social Group Bike Ride 1 to 3 hrs

Maintaining cardio fitness.

When your goal is to just maintain your current cardio conditioning (perhaps in the depths of winter), two rides with intervals during the week can be enough. One hard interval ride of at least one hour (interval time plus warm up and cool down) with four eight-minute LT/VO2 max combo intervals and one easy interval ride of at least 40 minutes (interval time plus warm up and cool down) with two eight-minute LT/VO2 max combo intervals. Done at the proper power levels, that would be enough work to keep your cardio conditioning at around its current level.

Maintaining Cardio Fitness – riding 2 days a week.

Monday	**Tuesday**	**Wednesday**	**Thursday**	**Friday**	**Saturday**	**Sunday**
Rest Day	Weights & Kettlebells	Bike 60 min with 2x8 min combo intervals	Weights	Weights & Kettlebells	Bike 90 min with 4x8 min 30:30 intervals	Weights

When you're in a cardio training, fitness building phase and riding a lot with a lot of intense efforts, your legs will tend to get sore. Very sore. When he's training seriously on his bicycle, Andy's legs often are so sore that just touching them can be painful. In chapter 6, on recovery, we'll cover the three basic approaches to handling soreness—ice, massage, and ointments. Using these will help, but you'll often still be riding with sore, heavy legs.

When our legs are sore, we tend to take it easy. It seems to make sense to give our legs some rest. But this is actually the wrong approach. A tip that Andy learned from a pro rider at a bike camp regarding sore legs really helped him. When your legs are sore, after a short warm-up, do a few short (10 to 20 seconds) but very hard sprint efforts in a big gear. Somehow these efforts alleviate the soreness and enable you to ride harder. Try it. It works amazingly well.

And, by the way, this also works well to alleviate soreness due to hard weightlifting sessions, hard kettlebell sessions, or any hard sports effort.

Evaluating your cardio fitness

So how do you know if you are in good cardiovascular condition? Here are some targets to aim at. These numbers are from data collected by Hunter Allen and Andrew Coggan and presented in *Training and Racing with a Power Meter.*

For men, VO2 max power of 3.5 watts or more per kilogram of body weight is good and is an excellent target for most athletes to aim to achieve. VO2 max power of more than 5.0 is excellent, over 6.0 is exceptional, and over 7.0 is world class.

For women, VO2 max power of 3.0 watts or more per kilogram of body weight is good and is an excellent target for most athletes to aim to achieve. VO2 max power of more than 4.0 is excellent, over 5.0 is exceptional, and over 6.0 is world class.

For men, LT power of 3.0 watts or more per kilogram of body weight is good and is an excellent target for most athletes to aim to achieve. LT power of more than 4.0 is excellent, over 5.0 is exceptional, and over 6.0 is world class.

For women, LT power of 2.5 watts or more per kilogram of body weight is good and is an excellent target for most athletes to aim to achieve. LT power of more than 3.5 is excellent, over 4.5 is exceptional, and over 5.5 is world class.

While these numbers are general targets, they give you an idea of how good your cardiovascular fitness is now and what you might choose to shoot for.

How to use your heart rate monitor

We have defined the intensities of cardio training in terms of power, but we haven't yet talked about how to use a heart rate monitor. A heart rate monitor can provide valuable feedback, but it is being relegated to a position of lesser importance and usefulness by the superior technology of power meters. Power meters are much more accurate because power is an absolute measurement. Heart rate varies with the intensity of the effort, and also with the ambient temperature, fatigue, recent meals, and our level of caffeination. It's an indirect measurement and thus much less accurate than using power. This is especially true for shorter efforts like VO2 max intervals because heart rate always lags behind effort.

When measuring your intensity, use power values. Your heart rate is a secondary measurement that can verify that you're working at the proper intensity and tell you how your body is responding to your efforts. For example, VO2 max efforts should push your heart rate to around 90 to 95 percent of your maximum heart rate. LT efforts should elicit heart rates of around 85 to 90 percent of your maximum. These are maximum heart rates during the VO2 max or LT efforts, not average heart rates.

If your heart rate is unusually high during intervals, the ambient temperature isn't high or low, and your meals and coffee intake haven't changed, the elevation of your heart rate could be a sign of excessive fatigue or incipient illness. It's a signal to ease up. If your heart rate is consistently low during intervals, it's possible that your VO2 max and/or LT have increased so that your power levels are now too low. This is a signal to retest.

A heart rate monitor can provide useful feedback on how your body is responding to cardio training. But it is much less useful in measuring intensities, so use it as a secondary measure. Your primary measure should always be power.

Your heart rate monitor can also help you track your cardio fitness over time. Say you've been doing cardio workouts four days a week for several weeks. How can you tell if your cardiovascular system is getting stronger? The best way to track how much stronger your heart and cardiovascular system are becoming is to simply track your eight-minute and 20-minute peak powers from your rides and races using power meter analysis software. Alternatively, you can retest. Do another eight-minute and another 20-minute time trial. As your fitness increases, both your VO2 max power and your LT power will increase.

The next best way to confirm that your cardio fitness is improving is to track your resting heart rate over time. First thing every morning, before you get out of bed, take your pulse. Record

> **Spinning.**
> Riding fixed gear indoor bikes following the lead of an instructor who has you do intervals by having you alternate pedaling harder and easier is called spinning. Spinning classes have become very popular in gyms throughout the country.
> While spinning can be a great way to work on your cardio conditioning, the problem is knowing how intense your efforts are. Are you working too hard or not hard enough? If you use a heart rate monitor, it can help you exercise at the correct level. If you do spinning classes, be sure to use a heart rate monitor.
> Spin bikes with power meters exist, but are rare because they're expensive. If you have access to one of these bikes, it's perfect. You can train precisely. An alternative that many bike coaches use is to have classes were each person brings their own bike with a power meter, a heart rate monitor and a trainer. Then everyone does the intervals that the coach specifies, but at their own correct power levels. This is also a great choice for indoor cycling.
> Go ahead and spin in a spin class, but make it as effective as possible by using at least a heart rate monitor and, ideally, also a power meter.

this number in your training log. As you improve your cardiovascular conditioning, this number will go down. Your resting heart rate is decreasing because the exercise you're doing is increasing the stroke volume of your heart by making the heart muscle stronger. A stronger heart can pump more blood with each beat so that it doesn't need to beat as frequently when you're at rest. How low can your resting heart rate go? Many athletes in aerobic sports have resting heart rates near 40 beats per minute (bpm). Andy's resting heart rate is right around 40 bpm. Top athletes like Lance Armstrong or Miguel Indurian have resting heart rates closer to 30 bpm.

A low resting heart rate indicates that your heart is strong. It also gives you a strong reserve capacity (the difference between your resting heart rate and maximum heart rate) so that when your body is stressed, it has the ability to respond without breaking down.

A low resting heart rate also says a lot about your overall health and risk of dying from heart disease. A recent (2010) study that tracked middle-aged adults for an average of 12 years found that men with resting heart rates above 90 bpm were twice as likely to die of heart disease as men with resting rates below 60 bpm. For women, the difference was more dramatic. Those with resting heart rates above 90 bpm were three times more likely to die of heart disease than those with resting rates below 60 bpm.

> A strong heart and flexible arteries are part and parcel of being and remaining healthy.

Other studies have demonstrated that those with resting heart rates below 60 bpm have a much lower risk of dying of cancer. Individuals with resting heart rates above 73 bpm had a 140 percent higher risk of dying of cancer than those with resting heart rates below 60 bpm. So what is the connection between resting heart rate and cancer? Researchers aren't sure, but think that your resting heart rate reflects your overall health. A low resting heart rate below 60 is an indication of good health, while high resting heart rates above this level are associated with poor overall health.

It's become increasingly clear that it's unhealthy to have a resting heart rate above 60 beats per minute. It's a sign of a weak heart and stiff arteries as well as overall poor health. In contrast, having a resting heart rate under 60 bpm is a sign of robust health. So you can see that it's vital that you work to improve your central cardiovascular fitness. A strong heart and flexible arteries are part and parcel of being and remaining healthy.

A note of caution for older trainees with low resting heart rates. Be cautious around doctors and in hospitals. Many doctors continue to believe that a normal resting heart rate is between 60 and 100 beats per minute. One of Andy's riding buddies went to a hospital with a minor injury. As part of his evaluation, he had a routine EKG. Within minutes, a doctor rushed in and insisted that he check into the hospital and have a pacemaker implanted as soon as possible. His age (close to 60) and low heart rate (high 30s) led the staff to jump to conclusions. He did not actually have a heart problem. Further tests confirmed this. He was just very unusually cardio-vascularly fit.

Because the medical profession rarely deals with the small portion of the population that's truly fit, many doctors come to the wrong conclusions when dealing with these patients. You need to let them know that you're an athlete. And be cautious.

Final thought about cardio training

We've laid out the basics of effective and efficient cardiovascular training in this chapter. Now it's up to you. You need to apply these principles and put out serious efforts consistently over time. If you do, you can achieve a high level of cardio fitness and keep it for the rest of your life.

Conditioning, Part 2 — Muscular Endurance

For a very long time, like many people (probably including you), we considered complete fitness to include cardio training plus weight training plus a little stretching to enhance flexibility.

This is still a very widely held belief. But this paradigm is missing a key concept. We had the endurance to go for hours at a good clip, and we were also pretty strong, but what we looked like didn't match our abilities. We weren't all that muscular. We also still had lumpy fat deposits at various places on our bodies.

To be totally honest, even after we abandoned the old fitness paradigm and found a better one, we still have some lumpy fat deposits (but they're a lot smaller now). We are also more muscular and our larger muscles help hide the fat. What does this tell us and you? In the real world, better doesn't equal perfect. It's just better.

> In the real world, better doesn't equal perfect. It's just better.

So what was missing? What did we need that would improve our body composition by building muscle and burning fat? That something—the missing key concept—turned out to be *muscular endurance training*.

Looking back now, it makes perfect sense. Strength training makes you stronger and improves your muscle tone, but doesn't do much to build muscle or burn fat. Cardio training burns fat, but it also burns muscle. This combo leaves you with less muscle and still carrying around extra fat.

What is muscular endurance?

Muscular endurance is that physical quality between maximum strength and endurance. It incorporates some of both. In a way, that makes muscular endurance a bit of a holy grail. It covers all aspects of your fitness at the same time.

We were introduced to the concept of muscular endurance by fellow powerlifters who were raving about kettlebell training. Yes, kettlebells are versatile tools. They can be used in many different ways. But they turn out to be totally unparalleled for developing muscular endurance, which is what will enable you to change your body composition. You'll be building muscle and eliminating fat.

> Kettlebells are totally unparalleled for developing muscular endurance, which is what will enable you to change your body composition.

Right now, you may be asking, *If developing muscular endurance is the holy grail covering all fitness bases at once, why not just work on that and forget about specific strength and cardio training altogether?* To tell you the truth, we (along with many other people) have tried this and concluded that it just doesn't work.

Why not? Two reasons, one mental, one physical. First, when you're working only on muscular endurance, you get really bored. There's no variety in the work, and it requires great mental fortitude to do the same thing several days a week on a continuous basis. On the physical level, the law of diminishing returns kicks in. You work hard, but improvements in your body composition level off and eventually stop. Your body needs variety, too.

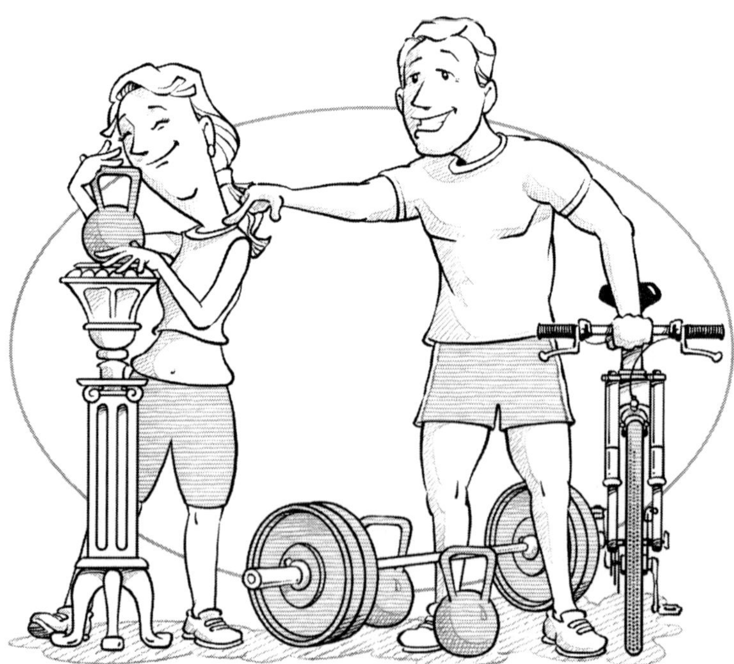

Don't fall in love with any one way of exercising –
your body and mind require variety.

If you're crunched for time for a few weeks because you also have a life to live, you can go ahead and work only on muscular endurance for a while. But be sure to return to a full training program when you can. This will keep up your strength and conditioning. It's a great alternative to quitting all training during the times when real life gets too busy.

How do you train to develop muscular endurance?

You train muscular endurance by doing high repetition sets of exercises using some type of resistance and taking short rest periods. This kind of training won't make you as strong as pure strength training will, but it will make you stronger. Similarly it won't increase your cardiovascular conditioning as much as pure cardiovascular training will, but it will increase your cardio conditioning. Muscular endurance training *is* unparalleled for improving your body composition.

So how do you do muscular endurance training?

It turns out that kettlebells are the ideal tool to use to implement muscular endurance training. If you're not familiar with kettlebells, they're like iron cannonballs with handles. Kettlebells are available in many different weights and sizes. The kettlebell is a versatile tool and can be used to perform hundreds of different exercises. With regard to muscular endurance training, however, we're only concerned with the handful of ballistic exercises that actually work muscular endurance.

Ballistic kettlebell exercises are exercises in which the kettlebell is moved rapidly for multiple repetitions. There are basically only three ballistic exercises, the swing, the snatch, and the long-cycle clean and jerk. We'll describe them in the following paragraphs. For muscular endurance training, any of these three exercises will work to produce results. The swing is the all-around exercise that does everything well. It's the basic exercise. The snatch and long-cycle clean and jerk, both of which require a much higher skill level, are very beneficial, but they require some

> Muscular endurance training *is* unparalleled for improving your body composition.

Kettlebell sizes.
Traditionally, kettlebells have come in three sizes—35 pounds, 53 pounds, and 70 pounds. As kettlebell training has experienced a resurgence in popularity, more sizes have become available. Starting at 5 pounds and going up to 108 pounds, many sizes are now common. This means that now everyone can find a kettlebell of the right size to train with.

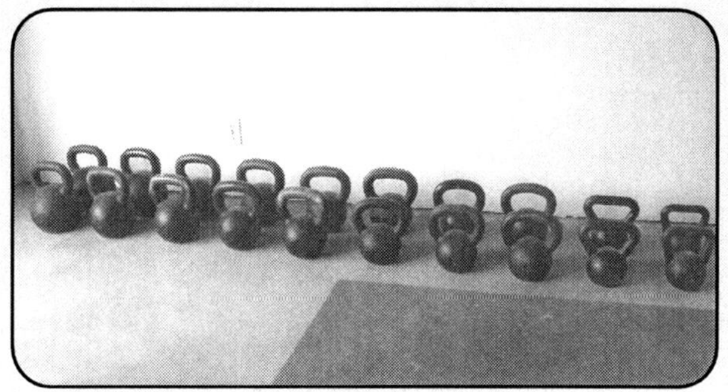

Kettlebells.

effort to learn and develop good lifting form. The snatch tends to work a bit better for increasing cardio fitness and losing fat, while the clean and jerk tends to work a little better to increase strength and build muscle.

How to perform the three basic ballistic kettlebell exercises

The swing.

Straddle the kettlebell and reach down to grab the handle with both hands by pushing your butt back. This starting position is the same as in the Sumo deadlift. Now swing the kettlebell up to chest height by snapping your hips forward. Your arms stay straight and are simply connectors between the kettlebell and the power generated by your hips. As the kettlebell comes back down, push your butt back. The power to move the kettlebell comes from the hip snap.

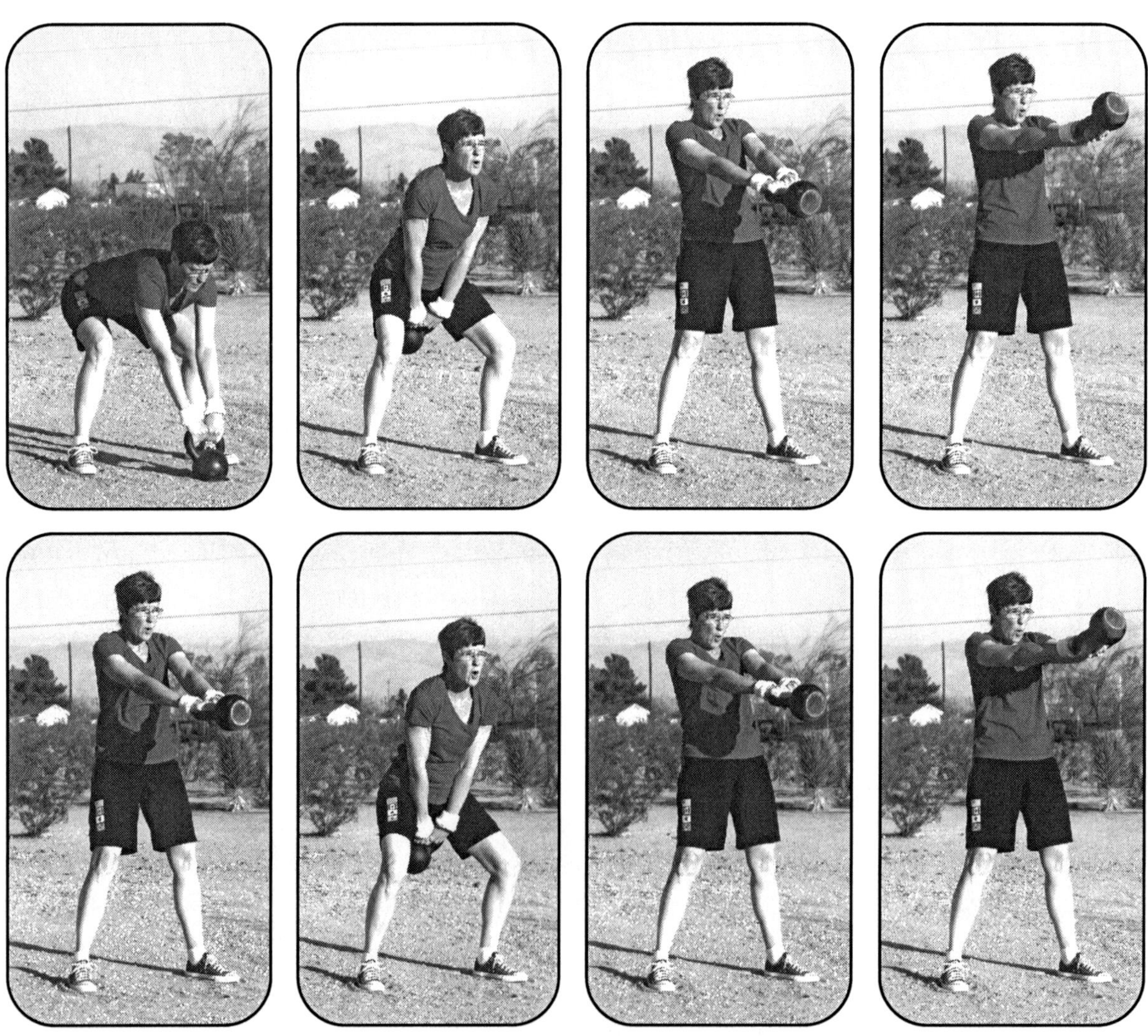

Swinging a kettlebell. The power to swing comes from the hip snap—the arms just connect the kettlebell to the body.

The snatch.

The basic movement is a one hand swing, except that when the kettlebell reaches chest height, pull it toward yourself using your back muscles, then punch your arm up so that the kettlebell ends up stopped over your head.

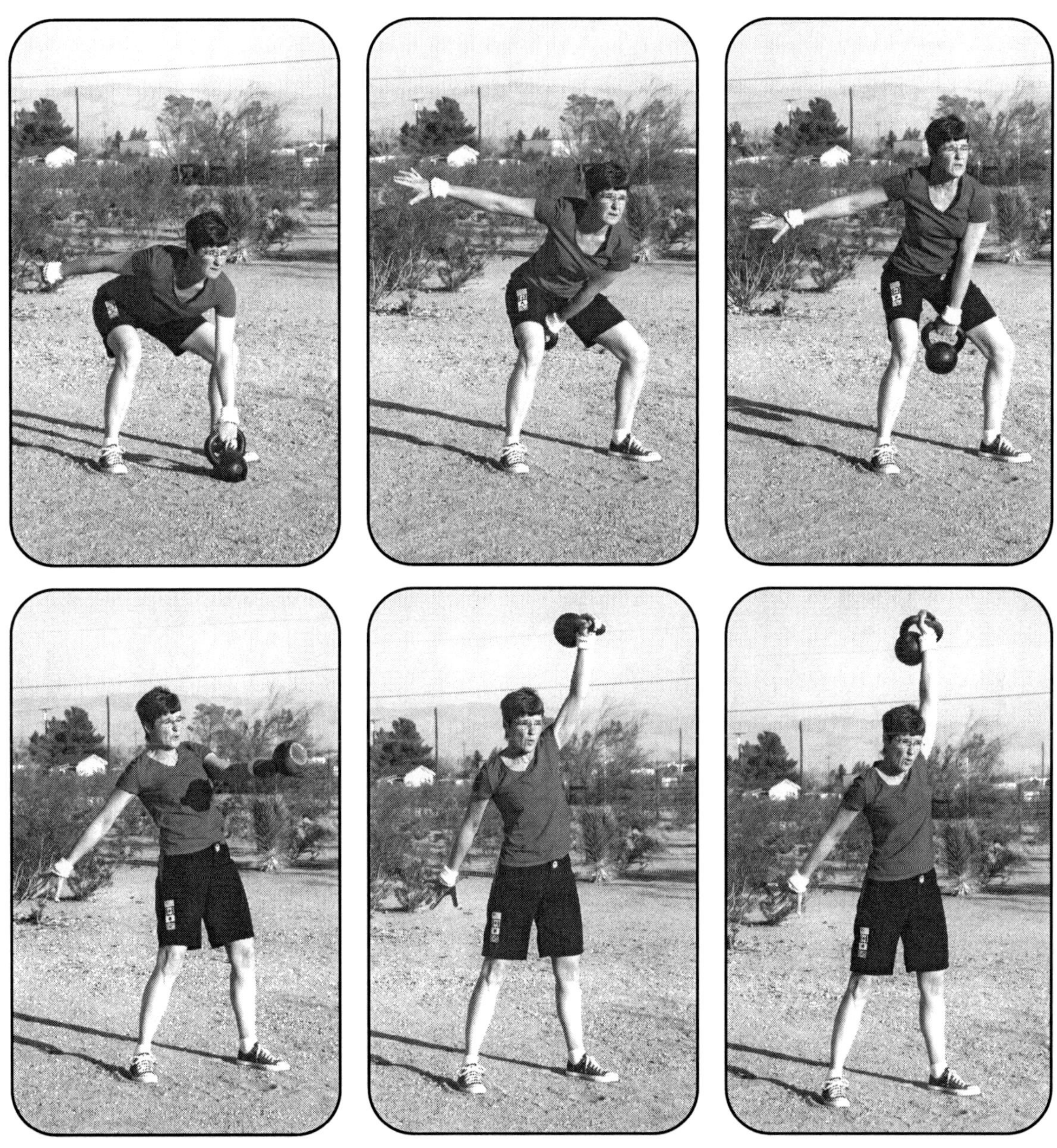

Snatching a kettlebell. It's a one arm swing with a stronger hip snap that projects the kettlebell overhead in a single smooth motion.

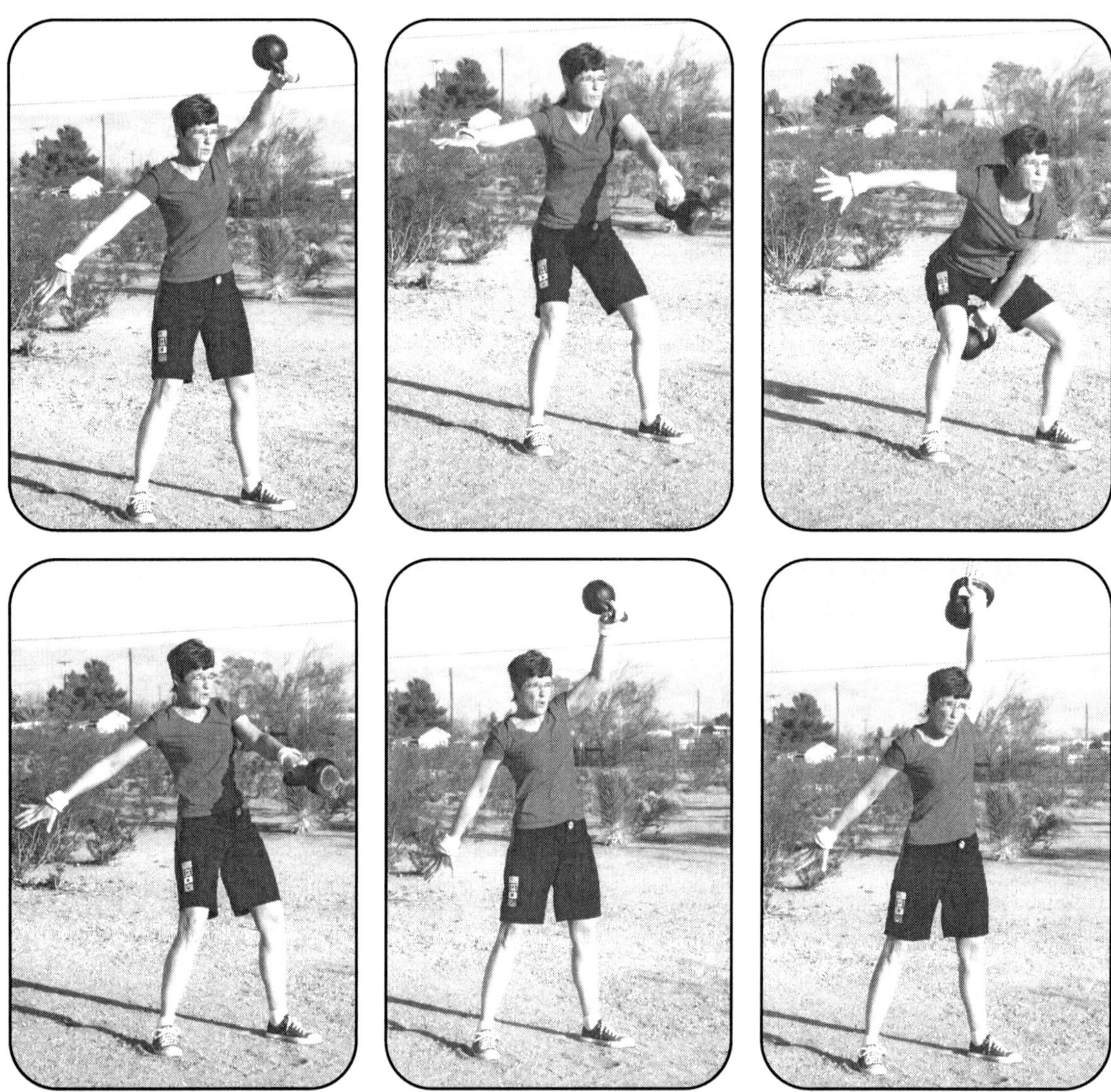

Snatching a kettlebell (continued).

The long-cycle clean and jerk.

This is a two-part movement. The clean involves bringing the kettlebell up to your chest by swinging it chest high and then pulling it toward you with the latissimus muscles of your back. Once it's resting securely on your chest, the jerk begins with a dip down by bending your legs slightly, then exploding upward. While the kettlebell is moving up, dip down again under the kettlebell and straighten your arm catching it as it stops moving upward. Complete the lift by standing up straight. When doing the long-cycle clean and jerk, you swing the kettlebell up to your chest before each time you jerk.

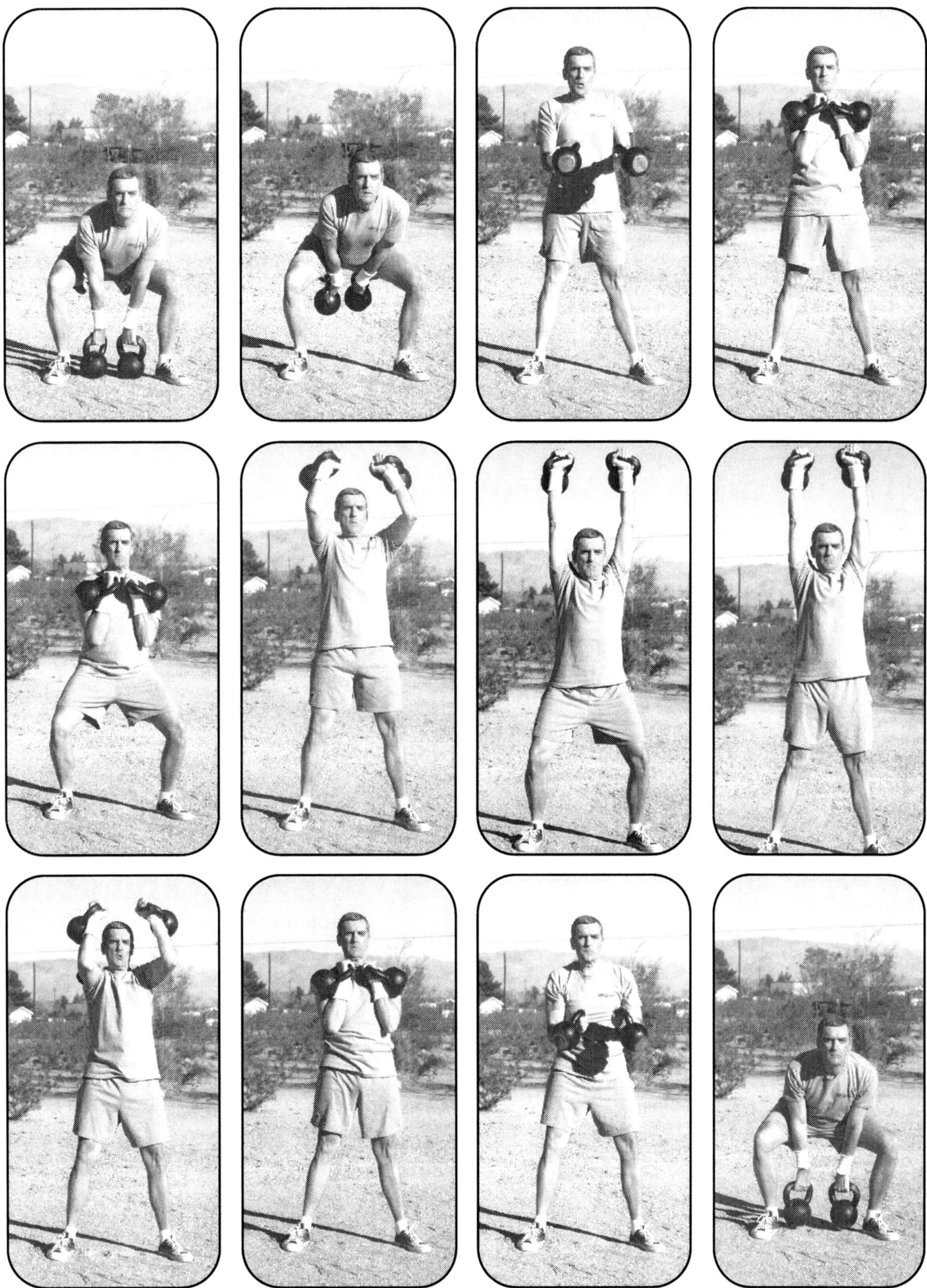

The kettlebell long-cycle clean and jerk is a complex series of movements that puts the kettlebell(s) overhead in the two phases.

It's difficult to teach these lifts with words and still pictures. Video is better, but still not all that good. Please seek out a qualified instructor to teach you these lifts. Russian Kettlebell Challenge (RKC) is the qualification we recommend that you look for. (Check www.dragondoor.com for a list of certified instructors.) Learning how to do these lifts right is absolutely essential so you don't hurt yourself. You'll be performing them for tens or hundreds or thousands and eventually millions of reps, and doing them right and safely is something that can't be overemphasized. Also, a qualified instructor will guide you as to what weight is appropriate for you in the different exercises.

> Seek out a qualified instructor to teach you these lifts. Learning how to do these lifts right is absolutely essential so you don't hurt yourself.

The movements are basic, but they work your entire musculature, plus your heart and lungs. Multiple high repetition sets with short rest periods will challenge your body in ways that it never has been challenged before.

How do you use kettlebells to train your body's muscular endurance?

The specifics for each exercise are slightly different, but the general principle is to do as many reps as possible in a set period of time.

What weight should you use? It depends on how strong you are, which exercise you're doing, and what your focus is. In general, if your primary goal is to lose fat, go with a lighter bell and do more repetitions. If your main goal is to build muscle, choose a heavier bell and do fewer repetitions.

> In general, if your primary goal is to lose fat, go with a lighter bell and do more repetitions. If your main goal is to build muscle, choose a heavier bell and do fewer repetitions.

For the snatch, most women should probably use an 18-pound bell, though strong women can use a 26-pound bell. Most men should probably use a 35-pound bell. Strong men can use a 44-pound bell.

For the clean and jerk, you'll ideally be using a heavier bell. For example, if you're snatching a 35-pound bell, you could clean and jerk with a 44-pound bell. That said, using the same weight can be productive, especially when first starting out.

For the swing you'll also want to use a heavier weight than you're using for the snatch. For example, a man snatching a 35-pounder could swing with a 44-pound kettlebell, or even with a 53-pounder. Again, work up to this weight and don't be afraid to swing a lighter weight.

The swing and clean and jerk can be especially effective in building muscle because the weight can easily be doubled by using two kettlebells instead of one. This gives advanced trainees the option to go even heavier to build even more muscle mass. But don't try to snatch two kettlebells at once. It can be done, but it can also be dangerous.

These are guidelines. When you work with your kettlebell instructor, you'll learn exactly what weights you should be using.

The swing

Let's start with the swing, which is the base movement for all kettlebell ballistic exercises. Don't underestimate its power as a standalone exercise. It works the entire body, and if you work hard and consistently, it will transform your physique. In fact, you may never need to learn how to snatch or clean and jerk. The swing alone is up to the task of training your muscular endurance to very high levels and in the process burning fat and building muscle to develop your body to its potential.

> The swing alone is up to the task of training your muscular endurance to very high levels and in the process burning fat and building muscle to develop your body to its potential.

The basic swing protocol is to swing for 36 seconds and then rest for 36 seconds. During each 36-second work interval, you do 20 swings. Swinging in this manner continuously for up to 35 sets will take just over 40 minutes (41:24 to be exact) to complete. But don't guesstimate the time. Use a stopwatch or timer.

A timer is a required tool for ballistic kettlebell training. It's just too hard to keep numbers in your head while you're exerting yourself hard. You can buy a low-cost timer that works from Gymboss ($19.95 at www.gymboss.com).

Let us tell you that swinging 35 sets nonstop is a truly Herculean achievement, both physically and mentally. For most people, even a fraction of that is an extremely hard effort. We've found that breaking the efforts up into seven-set blocks (just under eight minutes) with four minutes' rest between blocks makes it much easier to increase your workload up to a total of 35 sets than trying to do it nonstop. This modification makes it much easier to increase your total workload and makes it much less difficult mentally.

Why 36 seconds?

Kenneth Jay, a kettlebell master instructor and exercise physiologist, has studied effective training using kettlebells. From the literature of applied physiology and his own research, he has determined the optimum time periods for getting the maximum results from ballistic kettlebell training. See *Viking Warrior Conditioning* (Dragon Door Publications, 2010).

For almost everyone, the minimally effective dose of ballistic kettlebell training using the swing will be fewer than 35 total sets. If you're just starting out with muscular endurance training, one seven-set block will make a noticeable difference in your muscles and the amount of fat you carry. Working up to doing three seven-set blocks for hard (high-volume) sessions and two seven-set blocks for easy (low-volume) sessions will produce extraordinary body transformation. This is the goal we recommend for most people. For serious athletes of any age or for those truly motivated to be exceptional physical specimens, we push them to work up to five seven-set blocks for hard (high-volume) sessions and three seven-set blocks for easy (low-volume) sessions.

> If you're just starting, increase your workload slowly over time. You can start with one or two sets and work up to one block of seven sets.

If you're just starting, increase your workload slowly over time. You can start with one or two sets and work up to one block of seven sets. Then slowly add sets and blocks until you reach your goal amounts.

On your hard (high-volume) days, you need to push your volume up. Then on your easy days, do around 50 percent of the number of sets of your heavy day. For example, if you did one seven-set block plus one partial block of three sets, for a total of ten sets, on your hard (high-volume) day, then you would do one partial block of five sets on your easy (low-volume) day. Always round up any fractions. Thirteen sets on a heavy day would be seven sets on your next easy day.

Rest periods should always be 36 seconds within each block and four minutes between blocks.

We specify 20 reps per 36-second work interval because this tends to be the number of reps most people can do without compromising their form. Doing more than 20 reps at a time can lead to injury because of the extreme fatigue that some of the smaller postural muscles can experience. If you're just beginning muscular endurance training, you need to start with the number of reps that you can complete in 36 seconds while maintaining good form for every rep. This may be only 10 or 12 reps. Start there and build up over time.

When you're first starting to work muscular endurance with kettlebells, it is prudent to start with fewer than 20 swings in each 36 second work interval. Starting out with 10 swings and slowly building up to 20 swings is smart because it gives your body time to adapt to the stress. Remember that you need to push yourself beyond your comfort zone, but not into your pain zone.

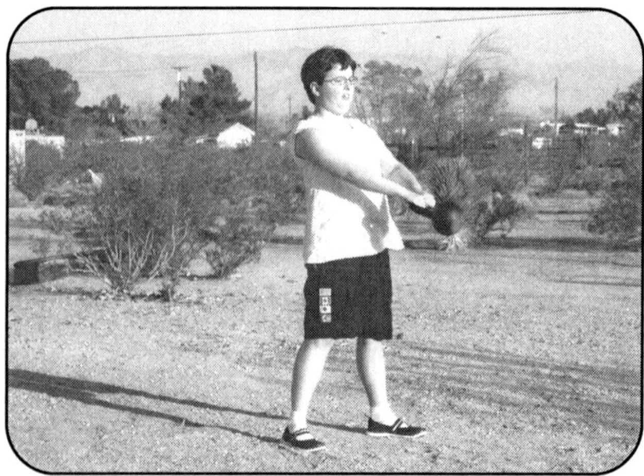

Our daughter Cori swinging a kettlebell.

Using only the two-hand swing, you can develop your muscular endurance to a super-high level. You can also create a transformation in your body with much more muscle and much less fat. It's intense, but safe and easy to learn.

And it's suitable for almost everyone. Even our daughter Corinna, who is both physically and mentally handicapped, was able to learn the kettlebell swing despite having difficulties with other forms of exercise. She works out with us and has become more fit despite her challenges.

> **Kettlebell training for handicapped individuals.**
> Physically and mentally handicapped children and adults face many challenges when trying to improve their fitness. Lack of balance, coordination, strength, and/or mental capabilities can all be roadblocks to doing the exercise needed to become more fit. Because of this, many handicapped individuals are in poor condition and as a consequence, their health and abilities suffer. Like the rest of us, they need to exercise.
> Muscular endurance training with kettlebells can help them get into better shape. With one easy-to-learn exercise (the two hand kettlebell swing), handicapped individuals can get stronger, improve their conditioning, and improve their body composition. See *Kettlebells for Special Needs Kids* at www.dragondoor.com.

The snatch

The snatch is a muscular endurance exercise that is unequalled in burning fat and developing VO2 max cardio conditioning. You don't need to learn to snatch to develop extraordinary muscular endurance because working the swing hard is sufficient to do that, but snatching is fun and can add variety to your training routine. It burns fat and develops your VO2 max a bit better than the swing.

The basic snatch protocol is to snatch for 15 seconds and then rest for 15 seconds. During each 15-second work interval, do five snatches with one arm, then switch arms for the next set. Do this continuously for up to 80 sets, which should take you just under 40 minutes.

Snatching like this for 40 minutes is even more of a Herculean effort than swinging. Very, very few people are physically and mentally tough enough to do it. Including us. So break the effort up into 16-set (eight-minute) bouts separated by four minutes of rest.

> **Why 15 seconds?**
> Kenneth Jay a kettlebell master instructor and exercise physiologist, has studied how to perform effective VO2 max training using kettlebells. From the literature of applied physiology and his own research, he has determined that this time period is optimum for getting the maximum results from ballistic kettlebell training using the snatch.

We specify five reps per 15-second work interval because this is the number that most people can do while maintaining good form. We also suggest that you start with a lower number of repetitions and work up. Also start with fewer sets and work up slowly, with the goal of reaching at least three 16-set blocks on your hard (high-volume) days. If you're particularly ambitious, you can work up to five 16-set blocks on your hard (high-volume) days, then on your easy (low-volume) days, cut the number of blocks to 50 percent of your hard days (always rounding up).

> Always build up your workload gradually. Your body needs time to adapt.

And always build up your workload gradually. Your body needs time to adapt. Even your hands need time to toughen up.

> To give you an idea of what world class conditioning is, let us tell you about a Danish Olympic athlete Mark Madsen, who competes in Greco-Roman wrestling in the 176-pound weight class. He was using kettlebell training for conditioning: 40 minutes of snatching doing eight reps every 15 seconds with a 53-pound kettlebell. He did the 40 minutes continuously. And he was doing this several times a week! This is a truly awesome performance and demonstrates what is possible by the truly elite athlete. We're telling you this so that you don't dismiss our suggested goals as impossible to achieve, which is what most people who start kettlebell training think, given that they typically struggle with doing only a few sets at the proper pace.

The long-cycle clean and jerk

The long-cycle clean and jerk is the kettlebell muscular endurance exercise that is unequalled in building muscle. "Long-cycle" means that you clean the kettlebell(s) before each jerk. You don't need to learn the long-cycle clean and jerk to develop extraordinary muscular endurance because working the swing hard is sufficient to do that, but like snatching, it's fun and can add variety to your training. And it can build muscle better than the swing.

The basic long-cycle clean and jerk protocol is to clean and jerk for 36 seconds and then rest for 36 seconds. During each 36 second work interval, do five clean and jerks. Working in this manner continuously for up to 35 sets will take just over 40 minutes.

But be aware that cleaning and jerking like this for 35 sets is very difficult. Because of the low number of reps, it tends to feel a bit easier than snatching or swinging, but even so, break the effort up into seven set blocks separated by four minutes of rest. As with the swing, each block will take about eight minutes.

Again, we specify five reps per 36 second work interval because this is the number that most people can do while maintaining good form. For most people, this will be five reps per arm using one kettlebell. As with snatches, switch hands every set.

Advanced trainees who want maximum muscle building stimulus can do the long-cycle clean and jerk with two kettlebells. This is much safer than two kettlebell snatches and the heavier weight will stimulate every muscle in your body to grow. And again, we suggest that you start with a lower number of repetitions and work up. Also start with fewer sets and work up slowly with the goal of reaching three to five blocks of seven sets on your hard (high-volume) days. On your easy (low-volume) days, cut the number of blocks to 50 percent of your hard day, rounding up any fractions.

Take care of your hands

Kettlebell training can be murder on your hands. The thick, rough metal handles, combined with the friction created by swinging and especially snatching, can lead to painful blisters and torn calluses. You will develop calluses that will protect your skin to some extent, but you need to pay attention to hand care. Blisters and torn calluses are painful. Worse, they will prevent you from doing strength or muscular endurance training until they heal.

That's why you must protect your hands. First, remember not to overdo. When you feel a tender spot, stop exercising and deal with it right away. Don't let it become a blister. Taping is the best protection against blisters, but it's impractical because it takes someone to do it for you who knows what they're doing. Find a gymnastics coach or a gymnast to teach you and a workout partner. A simpler protection that is almost as effective is a sock sleeve. Cut the elastic band off a pair of ankle-high socks and slip it over your hand so that it covers your palm. This works almost as well as a good tape job and is much easier to manage.

Calluses protect your hands, but if they get too thick they can catch on the kettlebell handle and rip off. Not good.

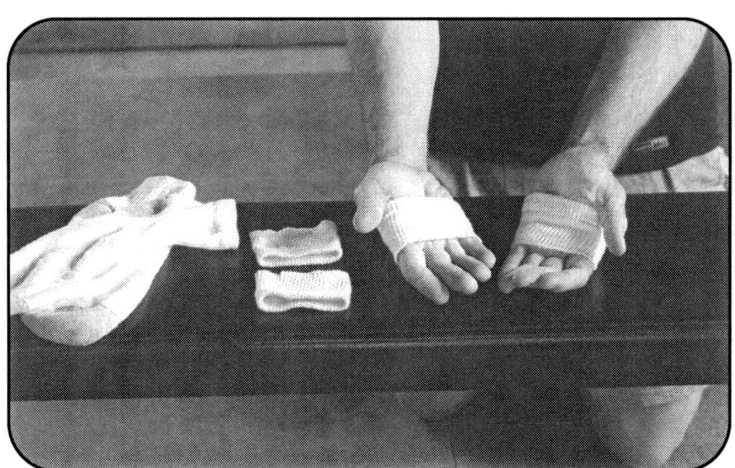

The sock sleeve – the easy way to protect your hands.

Next, control your calluses. Calluses protect your hands, but if they get too thick they can catch on the kettlebell handle and rip off. Not good. Use a callus file, light sandpaper, or a pumice stone to keep your calluses relatively thin. They need to be thick enough for protection, but not so thick they cause problems. This is a trial and error proposition, and unfortunately you will probably rip a callus at least once. Be philosophical. Consider it part of the learning process.

Finally, use a hand lotion that conditions your skin in addition to moisturizing it. Corn Huskers Lotion works well to accomplish this.

Realistically, how much muscle can you gain?

You need a realistic perspective of how much muscle you can gain when you're lifting kettlebells. For almost all of us, gaining muscle is difficult. Muscle is metabolically expensive to grow and maintain, and our bodies have evolved to resist having more than absolutely necessary. We're often misled by muscle magazines, personal trainers, and conventional wisdom. We're taught to believe that an average adult man can gain huge amounts of muscle in short periods of time. Typical is a friend of ours who started lifting weights with the goal of adding 30 pounds of muscle in three months to his average size, 5 foot 10 inch, 175-pound body. But that's just not gonna happen, not even with the assistance of steroids.

So *let's get real about muscle gains*. For example, let's look at Andy over the winter of 2009–2010. By Thanksgiving, he was winding down his bicycling (cardio focus phase) and getting ready for his usual winter strength and muscular endurance training periods. At the end of November, he weighed 160 pounds with 10 percent body fat and a lean body mass of 144 pounds.

> Gaining muscle is difficult. Muscle is metabolically expensive to grow and maintain, and our bodies have evolved to resist having more than absolutely necessary.

Starting in December, he did six weeks of strength training (Sumo deadlift and bench press ladders). He trained the bench press instead of the kettlebell clean and press because one of his goals for 2010 was to compete in a push/pull powerlifting meet. He then did six weeks of muscular endurance training (swings and double kettlebell clean and jerks). During this time, he ate a lot of pretty much anything he wanted, including plenty of protein.

By March 1, he weighed just over 170 pounds with 12 percent body fat and a lean body mass of just under 150 pounds. At first glance, working for three months to gain a mere six pounds of lean body mass would seem discouraging. In the real world, however, that's great progress in gaining muscle, especially for someone with a light frame. His wrist measurement (6½ inches) is the same as Michelle's, and she's a 5 foot 3 inch, 115-pound woman. Yes, Andy was really pleased with his winter muscle gains. He was ready to get back on the bike for his spring cardio training.

To help you understand how much muscle six pounds really is, go to the grocery store and buy six pounds of steak or a six-pound roast. Feel the heft of the meat. Check out the size of the roast. Now you have a better appreciation of what Andy achieved.

Or you can think about it this way. At the pace he'd set, he would add 24 pounds of lean body mass to his frame in a year. Of course in real life this just doesn't happen. If he kept doing strength and muscular endurance training without a break, the law of diminishing returns would kick in and his muscle gains would taper off and eventually stop. You just can't make linear projections like this in the real world. But thinking like this can help you appreciate the progress you're making. The bottom line is that this is an example of realistically achievable muscle gain. You can aim for this kind of gain. When you reach your goal, you deserve to be proud of yourself.

And keep in mind that in the winter of 2009–2010, Andy was 51 years old. Age isn't a barrier to gaining muscle.

Muscular endurance training — more of what you need to know

When you're training for muscular endurance, you need to focus intensely on swinging. For a change of pace and to slightly emphasize losing fat and building VO2 max cardio levels, you can snatch once a week. To tilt your training toward building muscle, you can do the long-cycle clean and jerk once a week.

But most of the time you need to swing. Do one hard (high-volume) session per week and one to three easy (low-volume) sessions per week. If you choose to snatch once a week, replace an easy swing session with an easy low-volume snatch session. If you do the long-cycle clean and jerk once a week, replace an easy low-volume swing session with an easy, low-volume long-cycle clean and jerk session.

When you're focusing on muscular endurance, you'll be doing three or four muscular endurance sessions a week. This is three or four swing sessions, one hard, and two or three easy. Once you're doing 20 swings every 36-second work set, further progress means extending the total workload up to either 21 sets, or 35 sets, depending on your goals.

Once you've reached your goal number of sets, you can consider increasing the kettlebell size. With muscular endurance training, the weight is less important than the total workload. If you can swing a 44-pound kettlebell for 21 sets, it's usually better to increase to 35 sets instead of increasing the weight to 53 pounds and dropping reps and sets swinging. It's often a judgment call, but if you can easily swing your current weight kettlebell for 35 sets, definitely go ahead and move up to a heavier bell.

The power of the kettlebell swing—from slacker to studette in seven weeks.

As a certified kettlebell instructor, Michelle needs to recertify every two years. This involves demonstrating that she can teach the proper technique in various kettlebell exercises. She also has to pass a fitness test, which consists of meeting chin-up and snatching standards. She is required to perform 100 snatches in five minutes using a 26-pound kettlebell. As anyone who's ever tried it can tell you, this is a very challenging test.

Earlier, she had reinjured her bad shoulder and so had not done any snatching for months. Now her recertification class was only seven weeks away. She was starting to feel a little panicky.

Enter the swing. She could swing with no shoulder pain, so starting seven weeks out, she did a combined strength and kettlebell workout every other day, which was three or four workouts a week. She leaned in to her once-a-week heavy swing workouts and worked up to 21 sets (420 swings). On her easier days, she did 14 sets (280 swings). Once a week, she did a very easy snatch session starting with 10 sets (50 snatches) and working up to 20 sets (100 snatches). This was to practice technique and give her confidence that her bad shoulder could handle the required number of reps.

Long story short, she was able to pass snatch part of the fitness test. (The chin-up part was a breeze.) The fitness test was a challenge, but thanks to the swing she was able to meet it in short order. Working the swing hard gave her—and will give you—a fantastic base of fitness that will enable you to reach all sorts of physical goals.

If you want to, you can do a snatch or long-cycle clean and jerk session for one of the easy sessions in the week. Follow the work/rest protocol to a comfortable stop. Again, use your judgment, remembering that this is an easy (low-volume session).

Here's the bottom line—when you're working to improve muscular endurance, your goal will be to set a new personal record in the total number of sets you're swinging on your one heavy, high-volume session each week and to complete two or three additional easy sessions of about half your high-volume session to boost the workload. You can substitute either an easy snatch or long-cycle clean and jerk session for an easy swing session, but you can get almost all of the benefits of muscular endurance training just by doing only swings.

> While snatching or cleaning and jerking can provide some variation and fun in your routine, if all you do are swings, you can still achieve very high levels of muscular endurance.

To use the swing to improve your cardio and cut fat, swing a lighter kettlebell for higher reps (20 reps per 36 seconds) and for more sets, up to 35 sets instead of only 21 sets. To emphasize building muscle, use either one heavier kettlebell or two kettlebells and swing for a lower number of reps (10 reps per 36 seconds) and for fewer sets (no more than 21 sets).

While snatching or cleaning and jerking can provide some variation and fun in your routine, if all you do are swings, you can still achieve very high levels of muscular endurance.

This muscular endurance training method we've presented here is simple and follows the 80/20 rule. It will produce excellent results in almost everyone. Remember, your ultimate goal is to increase your hard session swing sets to at least 21 with a challenging weight kettlebell. Working up to 35 sets will result in more improvement in your muscular endurance, but 21 sets will give you 80 percent of the results with much less work.

If you have specific strength and conditioning needs, you can modify your routine to customize the training and thereby further increase its effectiveness. For example, when she worked with mixed martial arts fighters, Michelle recommended that they work both the snatch and the clean and jerk to maximize both cardio conditioning and strength. She also suggested changes in the kettlebell routine to make it more specific to their sport. For example, fighters can snatch for three or five 10-minute bouts (five minutes of work) with one-minute rest periods between bouts. This mimics the three or five five-minute rounds with one-minute rest periods that they'll face in competition.

Similarly, they can clean and jerk two kettlebells for three or five five-minute bouts with one-minute rest periods between bouts. Instead of putting the kettlebells down during the five-minute bouts, hold them in the racked position. This is specific to grappling, where you're holding pressure and then need to explode to a new position where you again maintain pressure.

This example shows that although our programs are effective, they aren't written in stone. You can personalize and modify the specifics to improve them for your specific needs.

> **An added benefit—healthy joints.**
> In addition to being great for modifying your body composition, ballistic kettlebell exercises have the added benefit of being good for your joints. The movements, combined with the simultaneous impulsive loading of many joints, gently work your joints to strengthen them and make them work more smoothly. Many trainees have rehabilitated their damaged joints, especially shoulders and lower backs, with kettlebell exercises. See www.dragondoor.com for numerous examples. There is one caveat—you have to start easy and build up very slowly. Rehabilitation is a slow process, and it's easy to overdo it.

The effect of diet on body recomposition

It's vital not to forget the influence of diet on your body composition. Body recomposition is a two-step process of *exercise followed by eating*—and always in that order. Exercise, especially muscular endurance exercise, opens receptors on the surface of your muscle cells, priming them to absorb nutrients. When you eat after exercise, the nutrients go preferentially into your muscles instead of into your fat deposits.

Exercise plus more food (i.e., excess calories) results in building muscle. So to build muscle, you must eat more after you exercise. A lot more. Kettlebell training boosts your metabolism hugely, and building new muscles requires additional calories in addition to those required by your more active metabolism. Most people underestimate how much food they need to build muscle in conjunction with intense kettlebell exercise.

Extended bouts of swinging, snatching, or clean and jerking will boost your metabolism an amazing amount. After a session, your whole body will be not just sweaty. It'll be hot. It may take 10 to 15 minutes for you to cool down. This metabolic boost creates an afterburn that incinerates fat for many hours after you've finished a kettlebell session.

> Body recomposition is a two-step process of *exercise followed by eating* — and always in that order.

For example, when Andy is doing a muscular endurance phase using the swing and long-cycle clean and jerk with two kettlebells, he needs to eat like a lumberjack just to stay at his current weight. To gain weight, he needs to eat even more, enough, in fact, that he feels stuffed after most meals.

Note that when you take in excess calories after exercise, they will be shuttled preferentially to muscle. But some will still end up as fat. You cannot gain muscle without gaining some fat. Your goal is to gain as little fat as possible along with the new muscle. When you've reached your goal, you can reduce your food intake and lose that fat while maintaining most of the muscle you gained.

Exercise plus less food (i.e., a calorie deficit) results in losing fat while maintaining muscle. To lose fat, you must eat less after exercise. But not much less. As noted above, kettlebell training will boost your metabolism. You'll need calories. Cut back your calorie intake, but don't forget to eat after your workouts and include a pig-out meal occasionally to keep your metabolism up.

Note that when you take in fewer calories after exercise, they will be shuttled preferentially to your muscles. This means some of your body fat will be metabolized to make up the calorie deficit. This is how you can lose fat while maintaining your muscles. When you have a calorie deficit, you will lose some muscle mass. You cannot lose fat without losing some muscle, too. Your goal is to lose as little muscle as possible when losing fat. When you've reached your goal, then you can go back and increase your food intake and gain muscle with as little fat as possible.

> This is the simple secret to body recomposition. Exercise, preferably using muscular endurance exercise, and after exercising, eat.

It's a cyclical process. You move back and forth between gaining muscle along with a bit of fat and losing fat along with a little muscle. You can't do both at the same time. If you always just try to lose fat, you'll lose muscle too, which will lower your basal metabolic rate and make it harder and harder to stay lean. If you always just try to add muscle, you'll gain fat too and become pudgy. You must alternate back and forth.

This is the simple secret to body recomposition. Exercise, preferably using muscular endurance exercise, and after exercising, eat. Eat a lot or a little, depending on whether you want to add muscle or lose fat.

Accelerating your body recomposition

Americans tend to like quick results. We admit that seeing fast results boosts motivation like almost nothing else. So here's a way to accelerate your desired physical change and either lose fat or gain muscle.

Do some intense exercise before every (or almost every) meal. Keep a challenging swing weight kettlebell handy and do one set of 20 swings before you eat. This will prime your body so that the food you eat will be preferentially shuttled to your muscles instead of your fat deposits.

Doing these swings will also increase your weekly kettlebell workload. You will need to cut back your regular kettlebell workouts when you're doing this. Also remember that if you want to lose fat, eat less while you're following this program.

If you want to gain muscle, you need to eat more. For those bean counters who like to count calories, a rough rule of thumb is to eat 20 calories per pound of your lean body weight plus ten pounds. For example, if you weigh 165 pounds with 10 percent body fat, your lean body weight is 148.5 pounds plus 10 pounds, which is 158.5 pounds. At 20 calories per pound, this allows you 3,170 calories per day. But, really, you don't have to count calories. Just try to eat more than usual.

And don't lose sight of the fact that this technique is not a long-term training method. It's simply a way to see some fast results over two to four weeks. It will also give you the motivation to keep working on your muscular endurance.

Maintaining your muscular endurance

When you're focusing on developing strength or improving your cardiovascular conditioning, you need to maintain your muscular endurance. At these times, snatching or cleaning and jerking during your muscular endurance sessions is just too hard, both physically and mentally. Even if you only do easy (low-volume) sessions, these are the times when you only do swings. Try two sessions a week, one hard (high-volume) and one easy (low-volume) workout. Don't be looking to set a personal record. Swing at a comfortable level for you. Stretch, but don't push your total number of swing sets during your hard (high-volume) sessions.

The bottom line

Conventional wisdom tells us that you can't build muscle and lose fat with the same exercise. Kettlebell training defies this so-called wisdom. *It can actually do both.* And you can get the results you want by changing how you swing. If your primary goal is to lose fat, use a lighter weight kettlebell for more sets. If you want to build more muscle, use a heavier kettlebell with fewer sets.

You also have the option of adding in snatching and/or long-cycle clean and jerks to make your results match your goals.

The bottom line is that adding muscular endurance training to your physical training program will make you stronger, improve your VO2 max cardiovascular endurance, and improve your body composition by eliminating fat and adding muscle.

> Conventional wisdom tells us that you can't build muscle and lose fat with the same exercise. Kettlebell training defies this so-called wisdom. *It can actually do both.*

The past comes into the present

In the past, when physical work was required to survive, a man's muscular endurance was measured by how much he could carry and for how long. Try the farmer's walk. Pick up a heavy weight in each hand and carry it for as long as you can. Farmers carrying items such as full pails of milk gave this exercise its name.

Today, we measure someone's muscular endurance by how long and how fast and how heavy a kettlebell they can swing, snatch, or clean and jerk. Better than the farmer's walk, kettlebells measure one's muscular endurance ability. With kettlebells, you'll develop an iron hard body that is up to meeting tough physical challenges, whether in competition or recreationally. Or simply around your house and yard.

5 Putting Strength and Conditioning Together

The three qualities of superior fitness are strength, cardiovascular conditioning, and muscular endurance. All three qualities are needed. The challenge is that improving all three qualities at once is almost impossible, even for young, gifted athletes.

Even improving just two qualities at the same time is extraordinarily difficult. Realistically, you'll work to improve one quality at a time. Most people pick aerobics and work on only that, ignoring strength and muscular endurance. Not a good idea! Your fitness will be unbalanced. And if you ignore vital elements of complete fitness, it will be hard to make progress in getting fitter, even in the area you're working on.

> The real challenge facing anyone who is trying to achieve complete fitness is putting strength, cardio, and muscular endurance workouts together into a single integrated program.

So the real challenge facing anyone who is trying to achieve complete fitness is putting strength, cardio, and muscular endurance workouts together into a single integrated program.

The solution is to focus on one quality for one to three months while doing enough to maintain the other two qualities, and rotating so that all three qualities get worked over a period of several months.

Why one to three months? Because it takes at least a month to see some progress. More than three months, and you tend to get stale physically and psychologically and tend to plateau. The sweet spot is right around two months.

A good option is to match your program to the seasons. In midwinter and midsummer, when the weather is harsh, focus on strength development, which you can do indoors. In the spring and fall, when the weather is gorgeous and you want to be outdoors, ride your bike and focus on cardio conditioning. In between and for a change of pace, you can do a month or two of muscular endurance development working either indoors or outdoors.

The easiest way to accomplish working all three parts of fitness is to think in terms of exercise sessions. Schedule strength, cardio, and muscular endurance sessions. Plan each week by scheduling the number and type of sessions for each day. For example, you might schedule four cardio sessions on four different days of the week, along with two strength sessions combined with two muscular endurance sessions on two other days. Finish the week with one day of rest.

Studies have shown that you need only two sessions a week to maintain a physical quality as long as those sessions include some intense work. When you move up to three sessions a week, you start to improve the physical quality you're training. Moving up to four sessions a week creates substantial improvement. Five or more sessions will result in continued improvement, but at a much slower rate and with diminishing returns. For older trainees, especially, the return on more sessions declines quickly because of reduced recovery capacity.

Studies have shown that you need only two sessions a week to maintain a physical quality as long as those sessions include some intense work.

Using the 80/20 rule, you can see that four sessions a week gives you the best results for the time and effort invested. This is the sweet spot—the level at which you can make significant, noticeable progress. It's also reasonable and doable and allows for sufficient recovery.

Using the 80/20 rule, you can see that four sessions a week gives you the best results for the time and effort invested. This is the sweet spot—the level at which you can make significant, noticeable progress. It's also reasonable and doable and allows for sufficient recovery.

This is excellent news because it gives you time to do sessions to maintain the other physical qualities at the same time. This is critical because if you focus solely on one aspect and ignore the other two, you will regress and be constantly starting over in developing your fitness in the three areas. By working all three areas all the time, you can make progress in a smoother, easier manner.

The bottom line is that you need to focus on one attribute at a time for improvement. Schedule three or, ideally, four sessions a week for it and maintain the other two attributes with two sessions each per week. Every one to three months, rotate your focus to a different attribute. Over the course of a year you'll improve in all areas in a way that's both realistic and sustainable.

Seven or eight sessions a week means that you may be doing two sessions a day for one or two days a week. We strongly suggest that you double up two days a week to allow for a rest day or two every week. Recovery is vital. A rest day or two every week will definitely help you stay fresh.

For most people, it's easiest to double up the strength and muscular endurance sessions. You can do either a longer combined workout or split the sessions and do one session in the morning and one in the evening. Both options are good.

Given that each and every session needs to include some intense work, seven or eight sessions a week sounds challenging. But remember that the intensity will be an "I'm stretching myself" intensity, not an "I'm going to puke now" intensity. Also, only one workout each week will be difficult in terms of a high-volume of intense work. All of the others will include only a small amount of intense work.

How much of your time will all this working out require? This is a hard question because it will vary a lot depending on the person and on which fitness quality is being emphasized. Cardio workouts tend to require more time than strength or muscular endurance sessions. Generally speaking, you will need to set aside between four and eight hours a week to be able to complete eight sessions a week. That assumes about one to one and a half hours for each cardio session and one half to one hour for each strength and muscular endurance session. If your cardio workouts are longer, it could be more than eight hours a week. If you're working into a complete program, the time required could be less than four hours. Also, if you're working only to maintain fitness and not build greater fitness in any area, the time required will also be less than four hours.

Regarding the three or four workouts a week, if you want to improve the quality you're working, you'll usually have to do one session of a high-volume of intense work. The other two or three sessions will include some intensity, but only in smaller amounts. For the two sessions of the other two qualities you're not emphasizing, all of the workouts will include only a small volume of intense work.

Before you start planning your strength and conditioning program, you need to define your current status and what you want to achieve. Remember that you can't improve everything at once. Let's say that right now you have limited time and you want to lose fat and add muscle. As we wrote earlier, the way to accomplish this is to focus on muscular endurance training. Your strength development and cardio conditioning will be in the background and in maintenance mode at this time.

Training to improve your muscular endurance and body composition

A strength and conditioning program focused on muscular endurance would include three or four muscular endurance sessions along with two strength sessions and two cardio sessions for a total of seven or eight sessions per week. One muscular endurance session will be hard in terms of pushing to set a new personal record in the total time that you're swinging a kettlebell. The other two or three sessions will be easier. You'll swing (or snatch or clean and jerk) only half of your personal record number of sets but with the same weight and cadence.

In a full strength and conditioning program with emphasis on muscular endurance, you'll swing a kettlebell "hard" once a week. "Hard" means for more sets (higher volume) using an appropriately heavy kettlebell and the optimum cadence. You need to aim at setting a new personal record number of sets each and every hard workout. You may not be able to succeed, but that needs to be your goal.

> In a full strength and conditioning program with emphasis on muscular endurance you'll swing a kettlebell "hard" once a week.

The other two or three kettlebell workouts each week will be "easy," which means half of the number of sets of your last hard workout.

To maintain your strength, you'll do two strength sessions with kettlebell front squats and chin-ups. Because you're doing so much swinging (or snatching or cleaning and jerking) you'll want to give your lower back a break by not also doing Sumo deadlifts. You'll also give your shoulders a break by not doing any pressing.

Both sessions will be light in terms of volume (three to five sets of two reps) but intense in terms of weight used. Do these two sessions before two of your muscular endurance sessions. The strength sessions should be done on the same day as the muscular endurance sessions.

Complete your week by adding cardio exercise. Do two sessions on days that you're not doing any strength and/or muscular endurance sessions. Emphasize LT intervals because doing straight VO2 max intervals on top of so much snatching or swinging or clean and jerking (all of which work your VO2 max hard) is too much for most people. You need to do shorter sessions with two eight-minute LT intervals or two eight-minute combo intervals that include some VO2 max intensity. These sessions will work to maintain your endurance conditioning. And remember to include some VO2 max efforts every week.

Continue this weekly schedule for one to three months and work hard to increase the number of sets you're swinging in both the longer and shorter sessions. Watch your performance closely. If your progress is plateauing, ease up for a few sessions by reducing the number of sets in your hard and easy workouts, then push forward again. Remember that you're working to improve your muscular endurance. Keep focused on that goal. At the end of this one to three month phase, you should definitely be swinging for much longer than you were when you started. How much closer are you to that 35-set Olympic-level conditioning target?

Remember also that you're just maintaining your levels of strength and cardiovascular conditioning. In your strength training, don't increase the weights or volume. Use comfortable weights and stick to the prescribed reps and sets. It should feel almost too easy. Similarly, in your endurance training, keep your LT or combo intervals at your current power levels and don't try to push them higher. And don't increase the length of your bike rides, either. Keep the time very moderate.

This is the prescription for improving your body composition by reducing fat and building muscle and building overall fitness. *Remember that you need to work hard. Intensity is required.* It's not easy, but the results will make the effort worthwhile. If it were easy, you'd see a lot more buff bodies at the beach on your summer vacation.

The schedule given above is easily modified if your priority is to get stronger or to improve your cardiovascular conditioning.

Training to increase your strength

To emphasize strength, do three or four strength sessions a week. One heavy (three to five 1-2-3 ladders) and two or three light (two to three 1-2-3 ladders). Choose the Sumo deadlift and the one-arm clean and press with a kettlebell as your two exercises and definitely choose weights that are challenging. Test yourself every four weeks and adjust the weights upward as you get stronger. Alternatively, you can skip the testing, and once you can comfortably complete five 1-2-3 ladders for your heavy workout, just add three to five percent to your working weight and drop back to three 1-2-3 ladders.

Space your strength sessions so that your heavy day is not right before or after another strength session day.

When you set up your schedule for the week, space your strength sessions so that your heavy day is not right before or after another strength session day. For example, if you do your heavy strength session on Saturday, don't do another strength session on either Friday or Sunday. Do your two or three light strength sessions Monday through Thursday. Two sessions may be on back-to-back days, but that's OK because the sessions are light.

Make no mistake—doing three or four strength sessions a week is hard. But it's doable for almost everyone who works into it over several weeks. Even middle-aged and older trainees can handle the workload, at least for a few weeks. If you're not recovering after a few weeks, rotate into a cardio or muscular endurance period. In other words, do only a month or six weeks of strength building instead of plugging away for two or three months. As long as you come back to building strength regularly, you'll make much better progress with more shorter periods than fewer longer ones.

After two of the strength sessions, do some kettlebell swinging to maintain your muscular endurance. For most people, snatching or cleaning and jerking is too intense to add to lifting heavy weights.

Each week, do two light sessions at one half of your personal record number of sets of kettlebell swings. Add these muscular endurance sessions to two of your strength session days. Remember that you're just maintaining your muscular endurance, so don't push the number of sets up. You shouldn't work at more than 50 percent of your best. This should be enough effort to maintain, but not so much that you take away from improving your strength.

Now add two cardiovascular exercise sessions. Mix and match VO2 max, LT and combo intervals: two four-minute VO2 max intervals, or two eight-minute 30:30 VO2 max intervals, or two eight-minute LT intervals, or two eight-minute combo intervals. Always keep the intensity on both cardio days short, and don't try to push up the power. It's also a good idea to keep the overall time short. You don't want muscle fatigue to limit your strength gains.

This is how you get stronger. Work on it for one to three months. After this phase, you will be much stronger than when you started.

Training to boost your cardio conditioning

When you're working on improving your cardiovascular conditioning, you'll schedule three or four bike rides a week. Since you're only riding three or four times a week, you need to do something intense on every ride. Consider LT intervals or VO2 max intervals or combo intervals. One day a week, do a high volume of intense intervals four eight-minute LT intervals or four four-minute VO2 max intervals, or four eight-minute combo intervals. The other two or three workouts a week do intervals but for less total time two four-minute VO2 max intervals, or two eight-minute LT intervals or two eight-minute combo intervals. And don't get lazy! Always do some VO2 max intervals every week.

Let's do a reality check here. Facing having to work with real intensity on every ride can be very difficult psychologically. This is where terrain and/or other riders can be of immense help. If you're facing a hard ride with four eight-minute LT intervals, try a long climb. Work hard uphill at your LT on the steeper sections and recover for a bit on the flatter parts. This can make it much easier to accumulate 32 minutes at LT.

Similarly, on a group ride, you can go to the front and pull hard at your LT and then rotate back to recover, accumulating time at LT every pull. Like on a climb you'll do intervals of different lengths, but you'll reach your goal time at LT. This turns out to be much easier on the mind.

While you're working to build your cardio conditioning you'll need to do workouts that maintain your strength and muscular endurance. On two days that you're not riding schedule both a strength and a muscular endurance workout.

Two strength sessions a week will maintain your strength level. Because a lot of hard riding will leave your legs sore do kettlebell clean and presses and chin-ups. Both sessions will be light in terms of volume (three to five sets of two reps) but intense in terms of weight used. Do these two sessions before the muscular endurance sessions.

Follow each strength session with a light muscular endurance session at one half of your personal record number of sets of kettlebell swings. Remember that you're just maintaining your muscular endurance, so don't push the number of sets up. You shouldn't work at more than 50 percent of your best. This should be enough effort to maintain, but not so much that you take away from improving your cardio conditioning.

Just starting out?

Here's a good schedule to follow if you're just starting out with a focus on losing fat and building muscle.

- In week one, start with only two muscular endurance sessions per week.
- In week two, go to three muscular endurance sessions.
- In week three, go to four muscular endurance sessions.
- In week four, add one strength session.
- In week five, add a second strength session.
- In week six, add one cardio session.
- In week seven, add a second cardio session.

In the course of seven weeks you've worked into a complete strength and conditioning program currently focused on muscular endurance. Do the complete program for another week or two, and then rotate to emphasize a different physical quality

If you're starting out and want to emphasize building up your cardiovascular endurance and health you would follow a schedule like this.

- In week one, start with only two cardio sessions a week.
- In week two, go to three cardio sessions.
- In week three, go to four cardio sessions.
- In week four, add one muscular endurance session.
- In week five, add a second muscular endurance session.
- In week six, add one strength session.
- In week seven, add a second strength session.

Again, in the course of seven weeks you've worked into a complete strength and conditioning program initially emphasizing building your cardio conditioning and health. Do the complete program for another week or two, and then rotate to emphasize a different physical quality.

Finally here's a schedule to follow if you're just starting out and want to hone in on getting stronger.

- In week one, start with only two strength sessions a week.
- In week two, go to three strength sessions.
- In week three, go to four strength sessions.
- In week four, add one muscular endurance session.
- In week five, add a second muscular endurance session.
- In week six, add one cardio session.
- In week seven, add a second cardio session.

In the course of seven weeks you've worked into a complete strength and conditioning program initially focused on getting stronger. Do the complete program for another week or two, and then rotate to emphasize a different physical quality.

This break-in process will give your body time to adjust to the stress of a full program. And by starting out with the area that you're most interested in improving you'll be able to see significant improvement in that fitness quality that's most important to you. Seeing progress like this is tremendously motivating and will help you become consistent in your exercise program. This is vital in making exercise a part of your life and to seeing continued improvements in all aspects of your fitness.

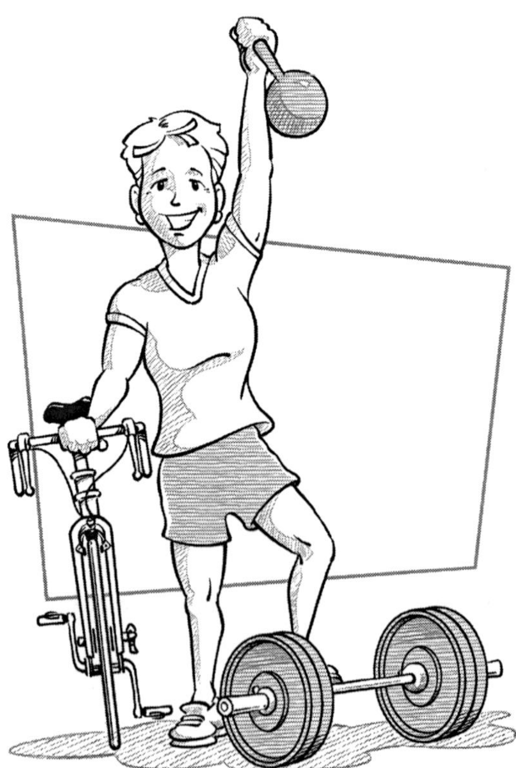

Absolutely, variety is necessary for complete fitness.

Your yearly plan

Now let's consider your strength and conditioning workouts over the course of an entire year. A balanced year might consist of two months of strength conditioning followed by two months of muscular endurance work followed by two months of cardio. Repeat this pattern twice to complete the entire year. Why two months? Because that's been shown to be the optimum interval that allows significant progress and avoids staleness. It can be shortened to one month or stretched to three months, but in the former case you make less progress and in the latter you risk reaching a plateau and even regressing physically.

> Consider your goals, priorities, limitations, and (most importantly) what you would like to do. *Achieving extraordinary fitness is just a matter of time.*

So now let's get real. Most people have goals and/or preferences. Plus real life—work, vacations, and other scheduled activities. And unscheduled things like getting sick. For example, Andy's priority is to enjoy riding his bike as much as possible. From April to June and from September to November, he does three-month cardio periods. From December to March, he does two months of strength training, followed by two months of muscular endurance training. Then in the heat of July and August, he does one month of strength work followed by one month of muscular endurance work.

This is not a balanced program. But it lets him do what he enjoys while still achieving complete fitness.

This is what you need to do. Consider your goals, priorities, limitations, and (most importantly) what you would like to do. Draft a yearly template that will work for you while also covering all of the strength and conditioning bases. *Then it's just a matter of getting to work. Achieving extraordinary fitness is just a matter of time.*

Measuring, tracking, and planning your fitness

Following a program that develops all three aspects of fitness will result in your becoming fitter. You'll be healthier, you'll improve your body composition, and you'll improve your performance in physical activities. Those results will be very apparent. You and others will be able to see them when you're playing a sport like tennis, participating in an activity like hiking, and when you wear shorts and a T-shirt in the summer. Your doctor will be able to see the results when he or she performs an exam.

However, these results are often anecdotal and difficult to quantify. Yes, they're real, but it's hard to put your finger on exactly where you are now and where you were before. Really, how fit are you now? How much fitter are you now than you were last year?

You have to measure your current fitness and track it over time. Keep track of personal best efforts over time. Keep track of personal best eight-minute and 20-minute peak powers on your bike. When you do this, your most recent numbers tell you where you are now, and you can compare them to your past numbers which will let you know whether you're improving, declining, or holding steady.

Also keep track of your personal best number of sets in the kettlebell swing. And your personal best weights in the Sumo deadlift, and the one-arm kettlebell press. Again, comparisons with past values show you where you stand.

These are all hard numbers and can't be fudged. They let you evaluate the results of your fitness program. They help you evaluate yourself. If you haven't been doing the work, the numbers will shine a harsh light on that fact. And if you have been working hard, the numbers will show it, reinforcing your efforts, and showing that your work is being rewarded.

Another way to measure and track your fitness is to calculate and follow your training load in each of the three areas of fitness over time. This method has the added advantage of enabling you to set goals for your level of fitness so you can reach a peak in fitness at a certain time in the future. This is invaluable for anyone who plays sports and has scheduled events and competitions. Or anyone who wants to be prepared for a planned adventure that requires excellent fitness, such as trekking Nepal.

Although the idea of training loads has been around for a long time, coaches and trainers have recently developed and extended this concept so that they can better track an athlete's fitness and readiness to compete.

When you're doing strength training, your training load is the total amount of weight lifted. It is equal to the weight times reps times sets for each exercise. For example if you do three 1-2-3 ladders in the Sumo deadlift with 200 pounds plus three 1-2-3 ladders in the one arm kettlebell press with 44 pounds, your total workload for that workout is 5,184 pounds.

Strength Training Load Calculation

Exercise	Wgt	Reps	Load
Sumo Deadlift	200 lbs	3 x 1-2-3 ladders = 18 reps	3,600 lbs
One arm KB Press	44 lbs	3 x 1-2-3 ladders = 36 reps (on each arm)	1,584 lbs
			5,184 lbs = total load

Similarly, when you're doing kettlebell training, your training load is also the total amount of weight lifted. Again, it's equal to the weight times reps times sets for the exercise(s). For example if you swing for 21 sets of 20 reps with a 44 pound kettlebell your total workload for that session is 18,480 pounds.

Kettlebell Training Load Calculation

Exercise	Wgt	Reps	Load
Kettlebell Swing	44 lbs	21 sets x 20 reps = 420 reps	18,480 lbs = total load

Thanks to power meter technology, it's now possible to accurately determine your cardio training load. It is simply the TSS (training stress score) for the ride. If you ride for 90 minutes with two eight-minute LT intervals, your workload will be whatever TSS value the analysis software calculates for you.

Your acute training load is the total for your most recent workouts. Acute training load is a measure of the physical stress and the level of fatigue currently being experienced by your body. Most coaches use the total load for the last week simply because it's easy to keep track of while also encompassing what you've been doing lately.

> Acute (fatigue) and chronic (fitness) training loads are intertwined.

Your chronic training load is the total of your training over a longer period of time. It's a measure of your fitness and ability to perform physically. Theoretically, it includes every workout you've done in your life, but on a practical level it includes only the past few months. This is because more recent workouts have an exponentially greater effect on your current fitness than workouts done many months or years ago. The most popular time frame for calculating chronic training load is seven weeks.

Acute (fatigue) and chronic (fitness) training loads are intertwined. The acute load will pull the chronic load up or down depending on whether it's greater than or less than the chronic load. And the chronic load constrains the acute load—if the acute goes too far above the chronic load for too long, the physical stress will become too intense and result in a performance crash. Top athletes and their coaches tend to calculate both acute and chronic training loads on a daily basis. When top performance is critical, this is what's required. For most of us, however, daily calculation is overkill. It just isn't necessary. Keeping track of our training loads can be very helpful, but we don't need that kind of precision. A good compromise between precision and ease of use is to keep track of your training loads on a weekly basis.

To calculate your weekly acute training load, add up the total workload for the week and divide that number by seven to come up with an average daily workload. If you want greater accuracy, you can use an exponential average that weights the most recent workloads more heavily than workloads earlier in the week instead of a simple average that weights all of the week's workloads equally. Your more recent workloads do have a bigger impact on physical fatigue than older ones. Nevertheless, the increase in accuracy over such a short period of time is not really worth making the calculation that much more complicated.

For example, let's say that you did two kettlebell session during the week—one with a workload of 5,600 pounds and one with a total workload of 10,560 pounds. Your total for the week would be 16,160 pounds. Your average daily workload would be 16,160 ÷ 7, which equals 2,309 pounds. This is your kettlebell acute training load for the week.

Kettlebell Acute Training Load Calculation

Kettlebell session 1	32 sets x 5 reps snatching a 35 lb KB	=	5,600 lbs
Kettlebell session 2	12 sets x 20 reps swinging a 44 lb KB	=	10,560 lbs
	Total training load for the week	=	16,160 lbs
	Av daily training load for the week	=	16,160/7
		=	2,309 lb
		=	kettlebell acute training load for the week

Now to calculate your chronic training load, you add up the weekly average daily acute training loads for the past seven weeks and calculate the exponential average. In this case, because of the longer time period it is necessary to use an exponential average load instead of a simple average. The more recent workloads have a much greater effect on your level of fitness than six or seven week-old workloads.

The formula for an exponential average is:

$$Ea = ((ATL - \text{previous week CTL}) * \text{smoothing constant}) + \text{previous week CTL}$$

Where:

Ea = exponential average

ATL = acute training load

CTL = chronic training load

seven-week smoothing constant = $2/(n+1) = 2/8 = 0.25$

For example, if your past week chronic training load was 1,462 pounds and your current week acute training loads is 2,309 pounds, your current week chronic training load is $((2,309-1,462)*0.25)+1,462 = 1,674$ pounds.

Note: To first calculate the chronic training load exponential average, you need seven weeks of acute training load values. Also, the first exponential average number will actually be a simple average value. As you add more values over time, the starting simple moving average will become a fully exponential average.

Once you've calculated your acute and chronic training loads, comparing the values can provide you with a lot of insight into your levels of fitness and fatigue. This is your training stress balance (TSB). Your training stress balance equals your chronic training load minus your acute training load (TSB = CTL − ATL).

To track your acute and chronic training workloads and training stress balance for your bike training, kettlebell sessions, and weight workouts, we suggest that you set up a simple EXCEL spreadsheet that does all of the calculations for you once you input your weekly workload numbers. It is also very helpful to graph the numbers to make them visual. Then it becomes very easy to follow the trends in your training.

Sample EXCEL spreadsheet keeping track of training loads

					Bike	KB	Wgt
3/27/11	tss =	240.0	ATL =		34.3	900.0	891.4
	kb lbs =	6,300.0	CTL =		31.1	1,350.0	1,122.9
	wgt lbs =	6,240.0	TSB =		−3.2	+450.0	+231.5
4/3/11	tss =	250.0	ATL =		35.7	1,500.0	1,337.1
	kb lbs =	10,500.0	CTL =		32.3	1,387.5	1,176.5
	wgt lbs =	9,360.0	TSB =		−3.4	−112.5	−160.6
4/10/11	tss =	280.0	ATL =		40.0	1,200.0	1,114.3
	kb lbs =	8,400.0	CTL =		34.2	1,340.6	1,160.9
	wgt lbs =	7,800.0	TSB =		−5.8	+140.6	+46.6
4/17/11	tss =	245.0	ATL =		35.0	1,342.9	1,142.9
	kb lbs =	9,400.0	CTL =		34.4	1,341.2	1,156.4
	wgt lbs =	8,000.0	TSB =		−0.6	−1.7	+13.5
4/24/11	tss =	290.0	ATL =		41.4	1,428.6	1,337.1
	kb lbs =	10,000.0	CTL =		36.2	1,363.0	1,201.6
	wgt lbs =	9,360.0	TSB =		−5.2	−65.6	−135.5
5/1/11	tss =	319.0	ATL =		45.6	1,071.4	1,000.0
	kb lbs =	7,500.0	CTL =		38.5	1,290.1	1,151.2
	wgt lbs =	7,000.0	TSB =		−7.1	+218.7	+151.2

(*Note:* this sample shows a time period focused on building cardio fitness by increasing the bike chronic training load.)

When your acute training load (ATL) is greater than your chronic training load (CTL), your TSB will be negative, indicating that your body is accumulating fatigue. But a negative TSB also means that you're pulling your fitness level up, so negative TSB values are required to improve your fitness. The trick is to pull up your fitness without fatigue that is too excessive for your body to handle. Generally speaking, this means negative TSB values that are not too negative. And it means not running negative TSB numbers for weeks on end. You need to run negative TSB numbers for one, two, maybe three weeks and then reduce your ATL so that the TSB value goes positive. Constant fatigue is bad for your body. You may increase your fitness over the short term, but sooner or later your body will break down and that fitness will quickly disappear. You need rest (indicated by positive TSB numbers).

However, when you rest, your fitness will start to decline. You want to hold on to as much fitness as you can while your body recovers. This means that you want positive TSB numbers, but not too positive. You can drop your ATL to zero, resulting in a very positive TSB value, but this will drop your fitness level very quickly. You don't want to run positive TSB values for many weeks because this will pull down your fitness level. You need exercise (indicated by negative TSB numbers).

> When you rest, your fitness will start to decline. You want to hold on to as much fitness as you can while your body recovers.

Do you see the pattern here? You want to bounce your ATL above and below your CTL in such a way that your CTL either increases or stays flat.

Graph showing bike acute and chronic training loads.

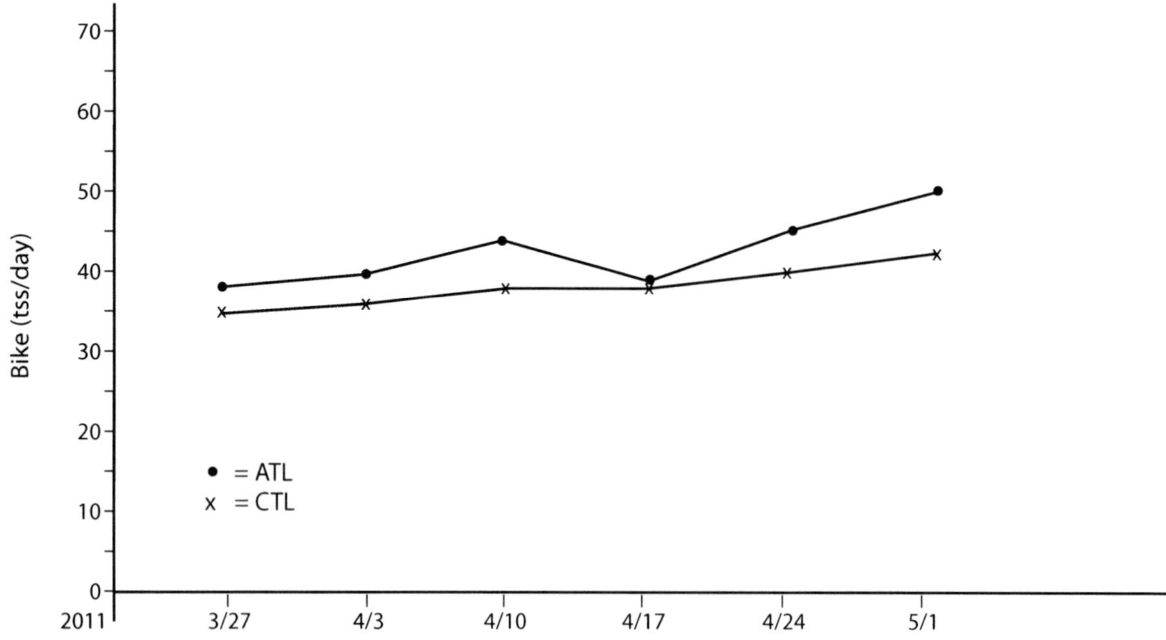

Graph showing kettlebell acute and chronic training loads.

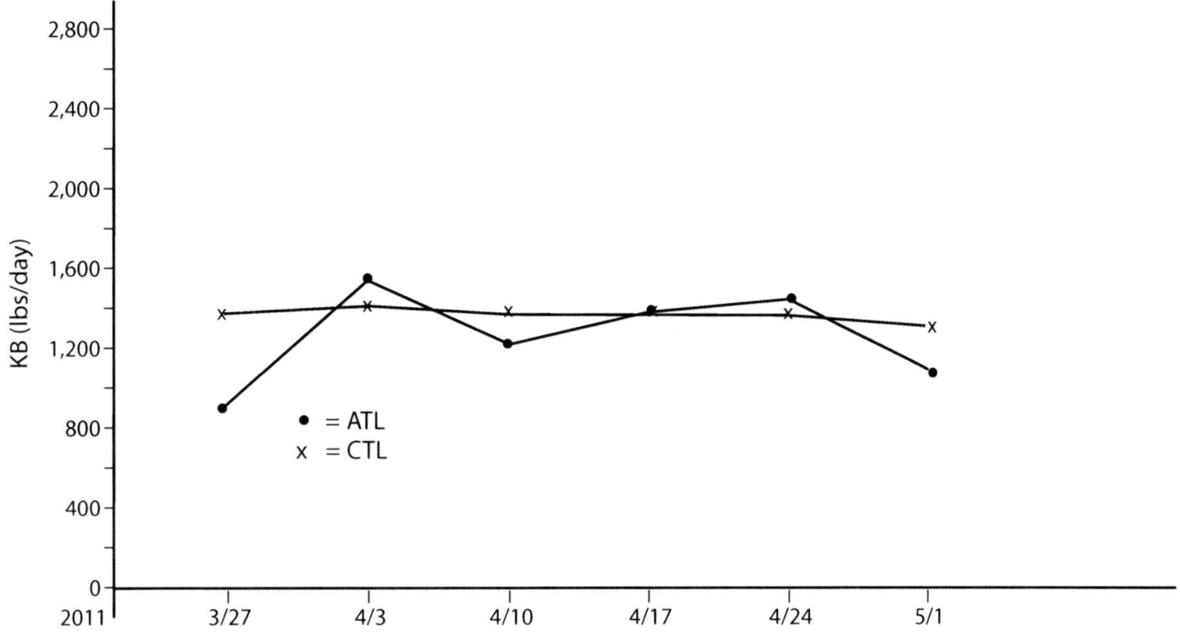

Graph showing weight training acute and chronic training loads.

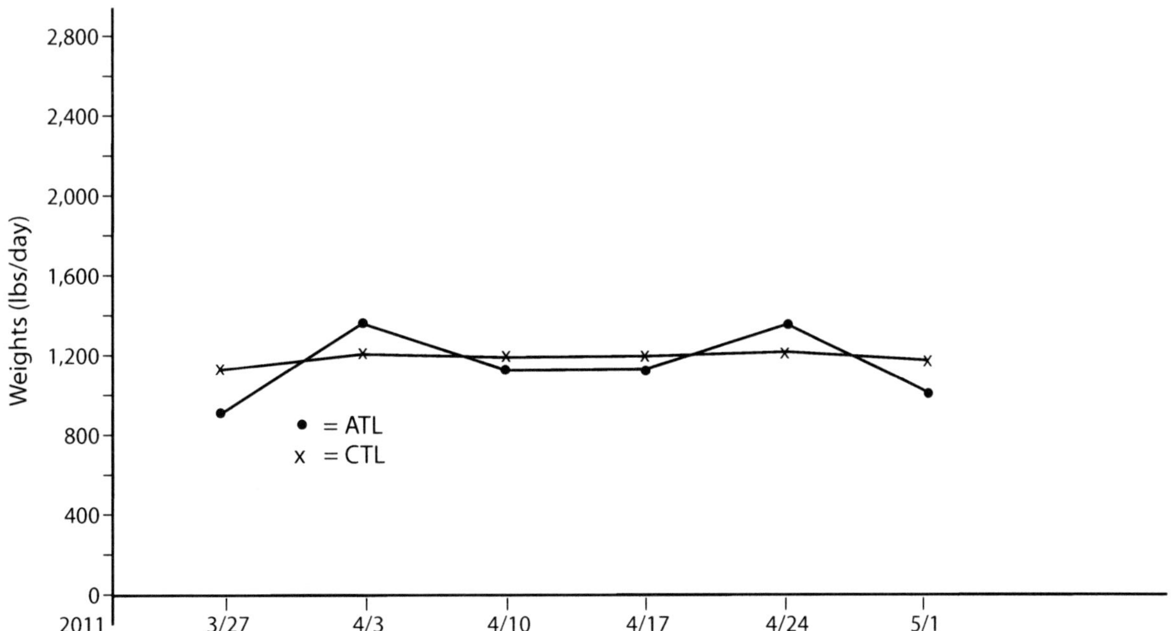

If you have an event coming up, it's important to note that your best performance comes after a period of high acute loads that have raised your chronic load to a high level followed by a period of lower acute loads that maintain the chronic load while reducing fatigue. This means that before an event, you want several weeks of negative TSB values followed by a week or two of positive TSB values that are just slightly positive. The result will be a high level of fitness combined with a low fatigue level, which is the recipe for top physical performance.

Now that you can quantify training loads and stress balance, you can also effectively and efficiently structure your training to pull up your fitness and peak for performance at precise times.

Putting the three training loads together for the three aspects of fitness

You want to schedule workouts that result in negative TSB numbers that pull up the aspect of fitness (strength, cardio, or muscular endurance) that you're working on. For the other two you want to maintain, you need to plan the acute training loads to bounce around the chronic training load, sometimes a little higher, sometimes a little lower so that your chronic training load (fitness) stays steady.

> Keeping track lets you see how hard you're working now (your acute training load) and see your fitness now (your chronic training load).

What is the value of keeping track of training loads? Keeping track lets you see how hard you're working now (your acute training load) and see your fitness now (your chronic training load). It also lets you compare the two (your training stress balance). Not only can you see all that, you can also plan future workouts to peak your fitness at certain times. And you can also compare to past values to find out how your current fitness compares to where you were in the past.

Tracking is an invaluable tool. We urge you to use it. It requires some time, but the ability it gives you to measure and track and plan all three parts of your fitness makes it time well spent.

A minimalist option

A minimalist option is a way to achieving pretty good levels of strength and conditioning. It's a shortcut in terms of sessions needed and time required, but you pay in terms of effort and results.

Work out three or four times a week. Do three to five sets of two reps in the Sumo deadlift and kettlebell one-arm press. Use heavy weights. Then swing a challenging weight kettlebell once hard, trying to exceed your previous best number of sets and two to three times easy for half the number of sets. The total time requirement each week will be less than four hours.

Doing just this much isn't even close to optimum, and your strength and conditioning will not be up to the level of someone who does complete strength, cardio training, and muscular endurance training. But it will take you a long way on the journey to superior fitness in middle age.

This is another perfect example of the 80/20 principle. This 20 percent program will likely put you 80 percent of the way to superb fitness. And it's better than what 95 percent of other people do.

You can always add more training later. A full strength and conditioning program will boost your strength and conditioning and muscular endurance from pretty good to great. In fact, you will eventually need to add strength and cardio conditioning workouts. Variety is needed to give your mind a break, and it's also needed to move past physical plateaus created by your body's adaptive capabilities.

6 Recovery – The Other Crucial Factor

Recovery is the yin to the yang of intense strength, cardio, and muscular endurance training. It is the second most crucial factor (behind intensity) for any trainee (especially any older trainee) who wants to achieve a high level of complete fitness. Recovery from intense training sessions is a major issue for all trainees. Recovery is critical to maintaining consistency and sustainability of any fitness program. Being tired and sore all the time degrades performance in all activities and makes life painful and uncomfortable. It's vital to focus on recovery and manage it just as carefully as your training program.

> Recovery from intense training sessions is a major issue for all trainees. Recovery is critical to maintaining consistency and sustainability of any fitness program.

This becomes even more important for middle-aged and older athletes. Even amazing athletes like Lance Armstrong, who came out of retirement to place third in the Tour de France, and Dara Torres, who qualified for her fifth Olympics in swimming at age 41, adapted their training to accommodate their need for more recovery time than they required when they were younger.

How to incorporate recovery into your exercise program

Typically, most currently recommended exercise programs include some type of detailed exercise schedule to give the body time to rest after stressing it with training. There are all sorts of schedules that are recommended to stress the body and then give it time to recover, adapt, and become stronger. Common examples include three weeks of hard workouts followed by a week of rest or specific combinations of heavy, medium, and light workouts over the course of a week. Exercise routines can quickly become complicated and confusing.

Through experience, we've found that simple workout routines are better. They are easier to implement, and work more reliably. How simple? Just alternate harder and easier workouts for whatever exercises you're doing. For example, if you're doing kettlebell snatches and you did 30 sets for your last hard workout, simply do 15 sets for your next, easier workout(s). Or if you did four four-minute VO2 max intervals on your bike today, plan on doing two four-minute VO2 max intervals during your next bike ride.

> The critical point to note here is that "hard" and "easy" refer to volume of effort, not intensity.

The critical point to note here is that "hard" and "easy" refer to volume of effort, not intensity. As a guideline, an easy workout needs to be about half the volume of a hard workout. If you're snatching, use the same weight kettlebell and the same number of reps during each 15-second interval, but reduce the number of sets by 50 percent. For VO2 max intervals, continue to do four minutes at 95 to 100 percent of your power at VO2 max, but do half the total number of intervals. When lifting weights, use the same weight, but do half as many ladders. This pattern of alternating hard and easy sessions works reliably, and is simple to figure out and keep track of. So leave complicated exercise schedules behind and just do this.

Don't forget about progress. During your hard sessions, you must push yourself to equal or exceed your last hard workout, but the next time, take it easy and give your body and mind time to adapt to the stress that intense exercise inflicts.

But don't become obsessive. If you've scheduled a light workout, but you feel strong enough to wrestle a bear and win, go ahead and ignore your schedule. Go hard and shoot for a personal best. Days like this are rare. Take advantage of them when they occur. But don't forget to take it easy the next time.

On the other hand, if you're scheduled for a heavy day but feel stressed out, sick, or weak, go ahead and do another easy day. But don't skip the workout altogether. Your body needs the consistency of regular workouts.

From time to time, you will find yourself doing several hard or several easy workouts in a row. That's fine. Your body isn't a machine. It needs some flexibility, not a rigid schedule. Stick with the heavy-light schedule most of the time, but be open to modifying it depending on how you feel.

Overtraining

A quick note about overtraining. You might think that, given the amount of intense training you'll be doing following this program, you'll be on the brink of overtraining all the time. What you'll learn is that intense exercise is self-limiting. If you try to do too much, you just won't be able to. Your performance will decline, and you'll have to train easy with low volume until your body adapts to the exercise you're doing and becomes fitter.

In the real world, overtraining is usually a result of too much exercise volume, not intense exercise. Riding your bike for four or five hours a day at low power levels or lifting light weights for many sets of 10 reps is much more likely to induce overtraining. If you follow the easy/hard rule, monitor your performance and adjust your program when necessary, you won't need to worry about overtraining.

How to recover better

Recovery begins by not overdoing training sessions in the first place. You need to train intensely, but only to the point of slightly exceeding what's comfortable for you. Unfortunately, many people have a hard time with this concept. They feel that to be effective and get results, they need to keep pushing themselves to the point of pain and puking.

> Recovery begins by not overdoing training sessions in the first place.

Having to push that hard is, of course, nonsense. Effective training need not hurt you. More importantly, *it must not hurt you* because otherwise the odds of your continuing to exercise are minimal (unless you have some serious masochistic tendencies). Being exhausted and sore all the time is a real bummer. If you dread your workouts, you're not likely to keep doing them. You'll change your schedule, then probably stop altogether. This concept is readily grasped by most women, but men seem to have a very hard time with it. In the real world, women seem to need encouragement to work harder while men need to be restrained from working too hard.

Recovery must be monitored during and after every exercise session. Since incomplete recovery degrades performance, it makes sense that the best way to monitor recovery is by monitoring performance. If performance is declining, recovery hasn't occurred, and you need to change to an easy session.

The reason you're not recovering is pretty much irrelevant. Maybe your last session was too hard. Maybe your stress at work has increased. Maybe you're not getting enough sleep. It doesn't matter what the reason is. When recovery is incomplete, you need to cut back on your training sessions to easy, low-volume ones. At the same time, if you put some effort into thinking about possible reasons for your incomplete recovery, you may be able to make some positive changes that will enhance your strength and conditioning training.

Here's an example from our life. In the months after our daughter was born, it became increasingly obvious that she wasn't developing normally. Many trips to the pediatrician were followed by appointments with specialists. Hospital visits involving painful tests were also on our schedule. Any parent knows the stress of seeing your child crying in pain and worrying about what kind of health problem they might have. This went on for many months.

During this stressful period, being able to exercise was one constant in our lives, and it helped keep us on an even keel physically and emotionally. But we weren't in any shape to exercise hard. It was all we could do to exercise at all. If we'd tried to exercise hard, we wouldn't have been able to recover from the added stress. So we did months of very easy workouts. Did our fitness decline? Of course it did. But at that point in our lives, being extraordinarily fit wasn't important to us. We were able to sustain a level of health and fitness that let us deal with the problems we were facing.

So in our experience, simply cutting back training by 50 percent when you need more time to recover is superior to using any of the complicated and detailed exercise schedules that seem to be so popular nowadays. These schedules are just too rigid. They don't take into account the countless factors that can affect recovery like stress, fatigue, nutrition, etc.

> Recovery must be monitored during and after every exercise session. Since incomplete recovery degrades performance, it makes sense that the best way to monitor recovery is by monitoring performance

When we measure performance to judge our recovery, we can schedule recovery (easy, low-volume) workouts whenever we need them and for as long as we need them. Training can—and should—be individualized. When you're feeling good, you can continue to make progress, but when you're feeling not so good, you can work easier for as long as necessary.

Here's another example of how to cut back when you're stressed. We live in the California desert, where the summers are brutally hot with temperatures well over 100° Fahrenheit every day. If we're outside a lot working or exercising, this heat puts extra stress on our bodies. We cut back our training in the summer and do mostly easy (low-volume) sessions so we don't put ourselves into a deep hole of excessive fatigue and declining fitness that will take a lot of time to recover from.

It's crucial to remember that when you need more recovery you must still continue to train. Skipping sessions destroys training consistency. But you must modify your sessions. Generally speaking, a recovery session is the same as a regular session except that it's shorter and has less volume. That is, the exercises are the same. The intensity in terms of weight, power or weight and cadence is the same. The rest intervals are the same. *But the volume is cut in half.* For example, if your regular session is 32 sets of snatches, your recovery session would be 16 sets of snatches. Consistency in training is vital, but since natural, unavoidable interruptions occur for every trainee for all sorts of reasons (such as business travel, illness, vacations, special occasions, etc.) adding additional breaks for recovery ruins training consistency and with that your fitness.

Most middle-aged adults have numerous responsibilities, such as kids, parents, work, civic organizations, etc., which often cause unexpected disruptions in your training schedule and add unforeseen stress that affects your training and recovery. You need an approach to training that can be adapted to your life circumstances as they occur. This is when easy, low-volume, short exercise sessions can be so very useful. You can squeeze them in and maintain that important training consistency.

Other ways to monitor your recovery

Tracking your performance is the best way to monitor your state of recovery. But there are other ways to monitor recovery that can also be useful.

Keeping track of your resting heart rate can let you know how recovered your body is. Count your heart rate for a minute every morning before you get out of bed. Soon you'll know what your usual resting heart rate is. If on a morning it's up by 10 to 20 percent, that means you're tired and need to take it easy. If it's up by 20 percent or more, it means you're exhausted or sick and need a day off. If you have an important competition or event coming up, however, such as a race or an important presentation at work, your heart rate will usually be up by 20 percent or more due to excitement and adrenalin.

> Keeping track of your resting heart rate can let you know how recovered your body is.

For example, Andy's resting heart rate is usually right around 40 beats per minute. If it's between 45 and 50 on a morning, he'll still work out, but he'll do an easy session. If it's over 50, he just takes a day off and rests. He understands that it does no good to stress his body more if it's already exhausted or sick. On the morning of a big race, however, his resting heart rate is often as high as 60. That's when he knows that it's just adrenalin and nerves, and he goes ahead and competes.

When doing strength training, your body often seems to have recovered. Your resting heart rate is about right, but the weights feel inordinately heavy. This can indicate fatigue of your central nervous system. Remember, you need to be fresh in body and mind to practice the skill of strength.

One easy way to check for central nervous system fatigue is to get a high quality hand gripper, like an Iron Mind Captains of Crush gripper (www.ironmind.com), that you can fully close only two or three times. Just after you get out of bed in the morning, pick it up and try to do a couple of reps. If you can't close it fully even once, that's a strong sign that your central nervous system is tired and needs some more recovery time. Work out easy today, preferably a low-volume cardio session on your bike.

How do you monitor your performance?

First, if during a strength or muscular endurance session you miss a lift, stop the workout. Record the time and how many reps you completed. Your session now becomes a recovery session with less volume of intense work. Try to go hard again at the next workout. What is a miss? It's when you can't pull the third rep in a three rep set of Sumo deadlifts. When you can't get your chin over the bar for a chin-up. When you miss a snatch. In most cases, it's pretty clear.

When you're doing strength training with weights or muscular endurance training with kettlebells, it's critical that you not go to failure. Don't keep going until you fail to complete a repetition. If you're not confident that you can make the next repetition, stop. Don't even try it. Going to failure interrupts the process of learning the skill of strength. It will make you weaker, not stronger. And going to failure with kettlebells risks injury—an uncontrolled iron cannonball falling near your body can be a dangerous thing.

What is a miss? It's when you can't pull the third rep in a three rep set of Sumo deadlifts. When you can't get your chin over the bar for a chin-up. When you miss a snatch. In most cases, it's pretty clear.

It's also important to monitor your performance while doing intervals on your bike. Using a power meter makes this easy. If you can't hold your designated power during the interval, your performance is bad. Stop the intervals at that point and ride home easily. Try again next ride after you've had some recovery time.

Here's a tip to help you monitor your bike interval performance even more closely. You can often tell whether or not you'll be able to hold power on the next interval during your rest period. During the rest periods, you need to keep your legs moving to keep the blood flowing through the muscles. The effort needs to be easy, about half of the interval power. If you have to stop pedaling entirely during the rest period, or you can't pedal at half the interval power, then you're getting too tired to do more intervals. Stop and spin home easy.

Use this information to monitor your performance during your intervals and rest periods. It'll make it easy to determine whether or not you're recovered. Keep in mind that accommodating to your need for recovery isn't copping out or compromising. It's smart training. The older you get, the smarter you need to train.

Ways to speed your recovery

Contrast promotes recovery, and doing a contrasting activity is more effective for recovery than complete rest. After a hard strength or kettlebell training session, your next session should be a cardio exercise session. This can be highly beneficial because aerobic exercise flushes blood through the muscles, which enhances their recovery. Alternating strength and cardio sessions really does help recovery.

Another point to remember is that proper nutrition has a huge impact on recovery. You need to consume enough food to feed your muscles so they can rebuild and grow. We'll go into detail on diet in Chapter 7, but we want to make one important point right here. Within an hour of finishing your workout, consume a large protein shake with creatine monohydrate. (We'll share our favorite shake recipe with you in Chapter 7.) Drinking a protein shake after intense exercise has been shown time and time again to improve recovery after training.

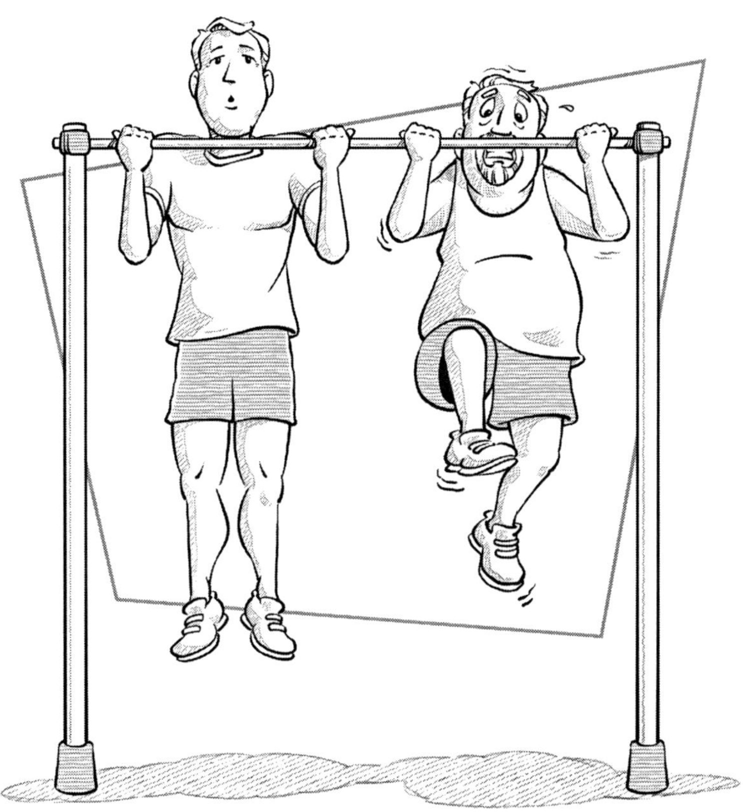

It's pretty clear when you miss a rep.

When you exercise intensely, you will experience sore muscles. This is normal. It's nothing to get freaked out about. Light aerobic exercise and some stretching (we'll talk a bit about how to stretch in Chapter 8) will help ease some of the soreness.

Almost everyone has some aches and pains, even without doing any intense training. The trauma that intense training inflicts on a body must be respected, especially if your body already suffers from some minor dings. (And who in the AARP crowd doesn't have any dings?) The best way to reduce inflammation from training and speed muscle recovery is to use ice on the afflicted area. Flexible ice packs are available at most any drug or grocery store and work well to cool inflamed muscles or joints. Or simply put some ice cubes in a Ziploc bag and use that. Or you can use a package of frozen peas or corn. Apply the ice for five to ten minutes. If an area is particularly sore, you can repeat the icing. But don't ice for more than ten minutes at a time; you want to cool, not freeze. Freezing can actually do more damage. Also, if putting an ice pack directly on your skin feels too uncomfortable, wrap it in a small towel. Icing sore muscles and/or joints after a workout is strongly encouraged. Two areas that are often sore, the lower back and the shoulders, are areas that can be iced routinely.

Anti-inflammatory drugs like ibuprofen can also be used to reduce inflammation and pain, but always after a session, not before it, or the pain that your body is using to let you know something is wrong and get you to stop before you seriously injure yourself may be masked. Remember that ibuprofen is a drug, not candy. Use it as directed and definitely don't use large doses because it can have nasty side effects like wrecking your stomach.

Massage can also work well in reducing soreness, but on a regular basis, it tends to be inconvenient and expensive. An option is self-massage. You can use foam rollers, stick massagers, and thera-canes. Doing it yourself is definitely not as nice as getting a massage from a masseuse or masseur, but it can be effective in resolving muscle knots and tightness and alleviating soreness.

Arnica creams also work well on muscle soreness. There are other pain-relieving creams, and we've tried a lot of them, but the only one that has really worked to reduce soreness is an arnica cream. A high-quality brand from Europe is Traumeel, which is fortunately available in the United States. Look for it on www.amazon.com.

You may have more than sore muscles. Joint soreness is an important issue. Knees, shoulders, and lower backs often become sore from the stress of intense exercise. If not dealt with, joint soreness can lead to injury. Moving the joints can help with joint soreness, and we'll tell you about joint mobility in Chapter 8. Anti-inflammatory drugs like ibuprofen are also effective in relieving joint pain.

But most effective in dealing with sore, inflamed joints is dimethyl sulfoxide, best known as DMSO. Pharmaceutical grade DMSO can be purchased in gel or cream form and is a tremendous help in reducing joint inflammation and pain. Don't be misled by people who tell you DMSO is an industrial solvent not fit for human use. In our experience, pharmaceutical grade DMSO works on joint pain safely and effectively. This is the high grade DMSO produced for veterinary use. You can be sure that million-dollar racehorses get the best treatment available, and that includes DMSO for their joints. One hundred percent DMSO can be very irritating to the skin, so we recommend a gel of 70 percent DMSO plus 30 percent distilled water. This is just as effective as pure DMSO and much less irritating. It's a better choice.

> Sharp pain in a joint may indicate an injury and needs to be checked out.

How do you distinguish between muscle pain and joint pain? Generally speaking, pain from sore muscles is located in the muscle and feels achy, not sharp. Sharp muscle pain is not soreness. It's an injury and needs to be treated as such. Joint pain can be achy or sharp, but it's clearly located in the joint. Sharp pain in a joint may indicate an injury and needs to be checked out.

A final point on aches and pains. Deadlifts, overhead presses, snatches, and clean and jerks strongly stress the shoulders, lower back, and other joints. This stress can lead to lasting joint soreness. What if you've tried the recovery modalities described above, but you're still sore? In that case, make substitutions like swings for the other kettlebell lifts and/or chin-ups and squats for deadlifts and overhead presses until the soreness resolves. This may take days or weeks or even months. You need to pay attention to how your body feels and adapt your training. Substituting exercises that are easier on your muscles and joints can aid recovery by reducing the stress on any vulnerable joints you might have.

A word about back pain

We believe that the kettlebell swing is superb in dealing with back pain. Because of injuries, Andy has experienced serious back pain since his twenties, but once he started doing kettlebell swings on a regular basis, the pain was substantially reduced. It returns occasionally, sometimes with a vengeance, but if he forces himself to get up and do some swings, he always feels better than if he just lies on the couch.

Others have had similar results. Kettlebell swings mobilize and strengthen the back, especially the lower back. This exercise can be used to rehabilitate back problems. Check out www.dragondoor.com, where you'll find several articles by physical therapists who use kettlebell swings in back rehabilitation.

Always use common sense. Pay attention to how much you do.

If you suffer back pain, be sure to have it checked by a physician. If your doctor clears you to exercise, try some two-handed swings with a light kettlebell. Sets of 10 to 20 reps several times over the course of the day will mobilize the spine, pump blood throughout the back, and strengthen the muscles.

Always use common sense. Pay attention to how much you do. Build the volume slowly. You, too, can get relief from back pain and improve your physical strength and conditioning at the same time.

Yes, it's counterintuitive, but working out is better for back pain than bed rest.

7
Diet and Supplements Are Important, Too

If you're an American reading this, odds are that you're at least a little overweight. An astounding two thirds of Americans are. This includes a surprising number of active Americans who, despite exercising, are still carrying five or ten or more extra pounds. And a large proportion of those people are on a diet right now. Although this is not a diet book, we need to talk about diet because unless you get your eating under control, attaining extraordinary fitness will be extraordinarily difficult, if not impossible.

There's been so much written about diet that we hesitate to add more. But when we look around in any public place in America today and see with our own eyes the rolls of fat most Americans are carrying around, we realize that something is very wrong. Most of those people don't want to be carrying that extra weight. Most of them have gone on one or more of the

> Diet strongly influences our performance and our ability to build muscle, so even if the amount of body fat you carry is not an issue for you, what you eat is an important component of your fitness.

popular diets advertised on TV or spelled out in any one of an avalanche of diet books. But even if they lost weight following current dieting conventions, they almost certainly soon regained it. Even those of us that are very active but are still carrying around excess pounds find that extra weight seems to be firmly glued to various parts of our bodies.

It's important to note that diet strongly influences our performance and our ability to build muscle, so even if the amount of body fat you carry is not an issue for you, what you eat is an important component of your fitness.

What can we add to the diet literature that might be helpful? A different point of view. We have an evolutionary perspective on what, when, and how much we should eat. We can also lend some common sense to your eating habits.

Almost all the conventional diet books and diet tips are oriented toward what you should and should not eat. This is an important issue, which we'll address, but we want to also cover two issues that are actually just as important—*when you eat* and *how much you eat.*

Before we get to specifics, let's examine the overarching principle that governs what a good diet for *homo sapiens* is. That principle is *evolution.* Over the last roughly 2.6 million years that hominids have existed and since the beginning of the Old Stone Age, or Paleolithic era, which is marked by the first appearance of stone tools, our bodies adapted themselves to the diet that was available. The diet of our prehistoric ancestors is what our bodies are still designed to eat. It's what promotes optimum health and function. We're going to address what, when and how much to eat, therefore, from an evolutionary point of view.

> We need to follow the principles of the hunter-gatherer diet for our bodies to work right and to stay lean and muscular.

Humanity evolved on the plains of Africa. Human beings filled the ecological niche of daytime hunter. Because they stood upright, early humans could see long distances. They sported a body covered with sweat glands but little hair, except on the top of the head to protect it from the blazing sun. All this enabled them to sweat and keep their body temperature cool in the daytime heat. These adaptations allowed physically inferior humans to prey on larger and faster animals. Animals covered in fur and lacking the ability to sweat couldn't handle the heat and had to slow down and rest during the hot African days, even while being pursued, whereas humans could track, flush out and chase prey at midday. The hunters came in for the kill with rocks or spears.

The hunters carried the animal carcass back to the small compound where they lived in small bands of relatives. The animal was butchered with stone flake tools and eaten raw or cooked over a fire. The meat and organs were shared, and everyone ate as much as they could. Anything not eaten almost immediately would be wasted.

Meanwhile, the women and children were collecting nuts, berries, roots, tubers, edible greens, insects, bird eggs, and other things that were side dishes when the hunting was good and survival food when it wasn't.

At dusk everyone gathered around the fire in a compound surrounded by sticks and piled thorn bushes for protection from predators. Their daily meal was freshly killed meat plus greens and the other side dishes. They went to sleep at dusk and woke at dawn to start another day.

This Paleolithic (Old Stone Age) hunter-gatherer lifestyle was how humans lived until the development of agriculture. The Old Stone Age was vastly longer than our modern agricultural age and lasted until the development of agriculture at the beginning of the Neolithic, or New

Stone Age, about 10,000 years ago. In evolutionary terms, 10,000 years is the blink of an eye. It's insufficient time for our bodies to evolve and adapt, so our bodies are still adapted to the hunter-gatherer lifestyle and diet.

Bottom line—we need to follow the principles of the hunter-gatherer diet for our bodies to work right and to stay lean and muscular. Fat, slow individuals didn't last long on the African savannah.

Fortunately for us, anthropologists and archeologists have studied ancient and modern hunter-gatherer cultures and learned how they lived and what they ate.

What to eat — the Paleolithic diet

In a nutshell (so to speak), our Old Stone Age ancestors ate meat, fish, shellfish, insects, eggs, fruits, vegetables, greens, and nuts and berries. Their diet was generally about 50/50 animal foods and plant foods. This of course varied around the world. The Eskimo diet was almost 100 percent animal foods, whereas the diet of Kalahari Bushmen was 80 percent plant food, though they didn't eat grains, beans, potatoes, dairy products, or sugar (except occasionally some honey).

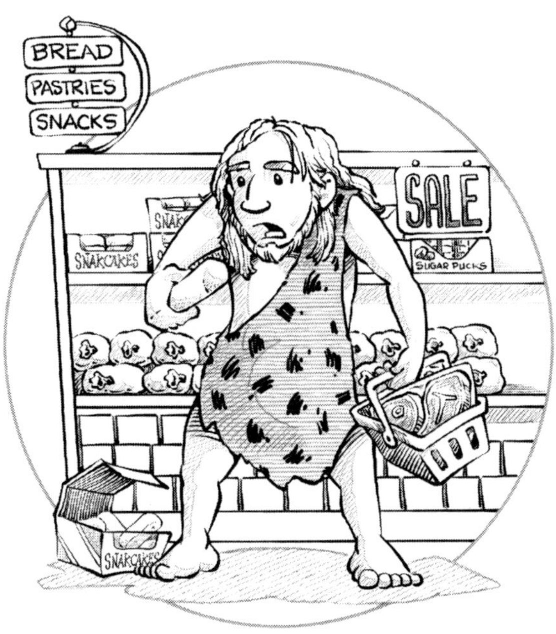

Huh?!

> At first glance, the paleo diet may seem restrictive, but it really isn't. There is a huge variety of foods that you can eat. For example, here's a recent typical day of eating by Andy. For breakfast—three hard boiled eggs and a sliced tomato (a little salt sprinkled on top of both), with black coffee to drink. For lunch—grilled chicken breasts and some stir-fried zucchini, with unsweetened iced tea to drink. After exercise, a protein shake (unsweetened applesauce plus water, whey protein powder, creatine monohydrate, walnuts and frozen blueberries). For dinner—stir-fried shrimp and asparagus, with wine to drink. All day, simple and tasty. And no counting calories. He ate as much as he needed so that he wasn't hungry anymore.

There are many books that describe the paleo diet. We recommend *The Paleo Diet: Lose Weight and Get Healthy by Eating the Foods You Were Designed to Eat* (Wiley, 2010) by Loren Cordain. In addition, there is a lot of information on the Internet about this diet. Yes, this diet is extreme, but extreme works—it's just another word for intensity. What most Americans are eating doesn't work. A big plus is that the paleo diet is simple. A few basic rules do the trick. Avoid eating any agricultural products made from corn, wheat, rice, any other grain, or any beans, potatoes, sugar, and dairy products. Do eat meat, fish, shellfish, eggs, vegetables, greens, nuts, and berries and fruits. Basically, you should eat things that our hunter-gatherer ancestors would recognize as food, but not eat anything that they wouldn't recognize as food. Of course, you can make it more complicated, but remember the 80/20 rule.

The paleo diet not only promotes health and physical performance, but it is also excellent for changing your body composition for the better by reducing fat and increasing muscle. How does it accomplish this? To explain, let's start with a little background on how our bodies work.

There are several hormones in our bodies that mobilize fat and one primary hormone that acts to store fat. That fat storage hormone is insulin. If you want to become and stay lean and healthy, you must control your insulin so your fat mobilizing hormones get a chance to work. Insulin, which is the key to fat control, is released whenever we eat. This release is vital to the proper assimilation of food. We don't want to stop the release of insulin. What we need to do is control the release so that it's moderate, not massive.

> If you want to become and stay lean and healthy, you must control your insulin so your fat mobilizing hormones get a chance to work.

How do we control insulin release? The first step is to eat modest meals. The larger the meal, the more insulin is released. A modest meal when you eat until you're no longer hungry will elicit a modest rise in insulin. A huge meal when you eat until you're stuffed will produce a massive insulin spike.

When you eat also has a major impact on insulin levels in your body. When we tell people that we fast every day, they tend to look for the vacant stare of some crazed cult member. But fasting for twelve hours of every day is easy. And it helps us control our insulin levels. If you eat dinner at seven p.m. and then breakfast at seven a.m., you've fasted for twelve hours. Your insulin has been controlled and it was easy since you were asleep for a good part of those twelve hours. For breakfast, lunch, and any snacks, eat small portions of low carbohydrate foods (except for your after-workout meal). Generally, make your evening meal your largest.

The most important step in controlling your body's insulin levels is to avoid simple carbohydrates—any white sugar or starch. A low carbohydrate diet equals less insulin release. Note that we didn't say *no* carbohydrates. Carbohydrates in the form of fruits and vegetables are perfectly good and are, in fact, healthy. When we eat whole fruits and vegetables we're eating a lot of fiber that blunts insulin release. Think about what your prehistoric ancestors ate. Meat, fish, insects, nuts and berries, vegetables, fruit, greens, and tubers. All low in carbohydrates and/or high in fiber. The principles of the paleo diet are what you want to follow.

> When you eat also has a major impact on insulin levels in your body.

All that said, there is a time to eat concentrated carbohydrates like bread, oatmeal, potatoes, rice, beans, or pasta (or even cookies and brownies). We eat these foods during the two-hour post-exercise window. This promotes the storage of glycogen in the muscles and liver. Glycogen is a form of carbohydrate stored in muscles and the liver. Muscle and liver glycogen is a rapidly available energy source when intense efforts are required of the muscles.

This is a modern-day exception to the paleo diet. Our Paleolithic ancestors didn't have concentrated carbohydrates available to them, so their bodies adapted to store more intramuscular fat and less glycogen. This let them work at less intense levels for longer periods of time, but their truly intense efforts were shorter and less frequent.

How important is insulin in determining how fat or lean you are? Obesity is a major risk factor in the development of Type II diabetes, and once you develop Type II diabetes, losing weight is one of the best things you can do to control it. Unfortunately, many doctors treat Type II diabetics by prescribing insulin (which we believe borders on malpractice). The result has been that patients treated with insulin were unable to lose any weight and many gained even more poundage, at which point their doctors would berate them for not following their diet. The reality is that if you're taking insulin, it becomes nearly impossible to lose fat because the insulin acts to encourage fat storage. A vicious spiral develops, with the patient getting fatter and having the dosage of insulin increased and then getting even fatter. At the same time, the patient's health declines quickly. This illustrates why it is so important to keep your insulin levels under control by manipulating when, how much, and what you eat.

To get as fit as possible, we're doing a lot of intense exercise and need more carbohydrate stores in our muscles and liver. To achieve this, we need to add concentrated carbohydrates to our diet at the times when our muscles and liver are depleted and primed to store those carbohydrates as glycogen. That time is after any intense exercise.

Our ancestors led more active lives than we do, with much more physical activity but less intense exercise. We modern athletes do much less total activity, but we ramp up the intensity to compensate. This difference is why we need those concentrated carbohydrates.

So following the paleo diet with the after-exercise exception lets us manipulate our hormones, especially insulin, to encourage our body to minimize our fat stores and maximize our amount of muscle. An added advantage to this exception is that it makes the paleo diet easier to stick with psychologically. You don't have to give up favorite high carb foods. Just eat them moderately after intense exercise.

The paleo diet in a nutshell.

DO EAT:	**DON'T EAT:**
Lean Meat (Beef, Chicken, Turkey, Pork, etc.)	**Grains** (Wheat, Corn, Rice, Oats, Barley, etc.)
Fish and Shellfish (Fish, Shrimp, Crab, etc.)	**Beans** (Black, Pinto, Lentils, Peas, etc.)
Eggs	**Potatoes** (white, red, sweet, yams, etc.)
Vegetables (Asparagus, Broccoli, Tomatoes, etc.)	**Dairy** (Milk, Cheese, Yogurt, Ice Cream, etc.)
Fruit (Apples, Grapes, Kiwis, Melons, Oranges, etc.)	**Sugar** (Sugar, High Fructose Corn Syrup, Candy, etc.
Nuts (Walnuts, Macadamias, Almonds, Cashews, etc.)	
Berries (Raspberries, Blueberries, Cranberries, etc.)	

Healthy vegetarianism?

We're not sure when it happened, but nowadays it seems like eating healthy is thought to mean eating a vegetarian diet. The conventional wisdom seems to be that if you want to eat healthily, you need to give up meat and eat only grains, vegetables, and fruit.

Let's not beat around the bush. This is just plain WRONG. Humans did not evolve eating only plant foods, and especially not grains and beans, which are products of modern agriculture. Humans evolved eating animals. In fact, many scientists hypothesize that eating animals was a critical factor that drove hominids to evolve into modern humans. The concentrated calories and nutrients in the meat, fat, and organs facilitated the development of our large, energy-consuming brains. Humans do best on a diet that includes a substantial proportion of animal products. A healthy diet is a meat-rich diet. It's vegetarian diets that are in reality unhealthy.

Supporting the fact that a vegetarian diet is evolutionarily wrong for humans is research done by Loren Cordain. Studying hunter-gatherers he evaluated the diet of 229 different groups and found that not a single one had a vegetarian diet.

How much to eat?

Now let's talk about *how much* you eat. If you weigh more than you should, you eat too much. Harsh, but true. It's too easy to overeat. The other day we took our kids to McDonalds as a special treat. (Our son had just graduated from middle school and chose Mickey D's for lunch.) Andy is not a big guy (5'10" tall, and 165 pounds), but he was hungry and easily scarfed down two Quarter Pounders, a medium order of fries, and a medium Coke. When we checked the nutritional information later, we were shocked. Each of those Quarter Pounders was just over 500 calories and the fries and Coke combined to add an additional 600 calories. Andy ate a grand total of over 1,600 calories for lunch—more than half of his daily caloric requirement. Add breakfast and a larger dinner, along with a snack or two, and the calorie total is way more than he needed for the day. If he ate like this every day, he'd get fat pretty darn quick.

And that's the point—a lot of Americans do eat like this every day. And even if you don't eat fast food, you eat three larger meals and a couple of snacks every day. That's the recipe for obesity.

Bottom line—YOU NEED TO EAT LESS. And to eat less, you must come to grips with hunger. A lot of people seem to think that if you miss a meal and your belly starts to growl a bit, you'll keel over from starvation any second. The truth is that feeling hungry won't hurt you. It can actually help you if you use it. Hunger can make the food you eat more appealing and satisfying. It can also tell you when to stop eating.

Eat until you're no longer hungry rather than until you're full. This is a fine distinction, but a hugely important one. Eating until you feel full is eating too much. Eating until your hunger is gone is eating enough. The rub is that if you aren't hungry when you start to eat, you won't be able to tell when your hunger is sated. You need to be hungry as a signal when to eat and when to stop eating.

How to eat less? Try to develop a few meals that you like, are easy to prepare, and follow the principles of the paleo diet. Then eat these same meals over and over again. Then you won't need to be continually deciding what to eat, and the boredom of a repetitive menu will help you to not overeat. Use this handful of recipes for 80 percent of your meals and then eat whatever you want for the other 20 percent.

> Eat until you're no longer hungry rather than until you're full.

Do not drink calories. Drink as much as you want of plain water, unsweetened tea, black coffee, or any other drink without calories, but do not drink soft drinks or fruit juices or milk. We make an exception to this rule for wine and beer, which are two of life's great pleasures … we can't imagine an enjoyable life without them. But drink moderately with the realization that beer and wine do indeed contribute to your caloric intake. The good news is that water, tea, coffee, wine, and beer are all beverages that are healthy for you.

And even though alcohol is high in calories (7.5 calories per gram, almost as much as fat), it doesn't appear to promote obesity. A study of 160,000 people over a five year period showed that those who regularly and frequently drank alcohol were LESS likely to experience an increase in waist circumference.[3] This means you can go ahead and enjoy drinking beer and/or wine without any guilt.

Having said all that about eating less, we need to mention that overeating can be good. Sometimes. Anyone who's ever been on a diet knows that the body is smart. The human body is a wonder of evolution. If the body senses that food is scarce, it down-regulates its metabolism and hoards fat to prevent starvation. This increases your odds of survival during famine, a situation that was common in the past. But nowadays this metabolic down-regulation just results in your quickly regaining all of the weight you lost while dieting … and maybe adding more when you stop dieting and return to your normal level of food consumption. Of course, part of the diet solution is to realize that you need to embrace a new normal. Your eating habits need to change for the long term.

Our Paleolithic ancestors were forced into this pattern of eating. Most of the time back then, food was scarce and there was only enough to stave off a little bit of their hunger. That's why they gorged after a successful hunt. They ate not until they were just full but until they were stuffed.

---

[3] *BBC News,* April 17, 2009. *American Journal of Clinical Nutrition,* 87:957-963, 2008.

The upshot is that today we need to eat less, though every once in a while we still need to pig out. That's great news! You can go out and eat whatever you want and crave, and you can eat as much of it as you can stomach. The not so great news is that you can only do this occasionally.

How occasionally? It depends. If you're at a good weight for yourself you can follow the 80/20 rule. Eighty percent of your meals should be controlled, and 20 percent can be open to whatever you want to eat. If you need to lose the weight, you might need to watch what you eat a little closer, but then you can return to 80/20 percent to maintain your weight. The bottom line is that most of the time you need to eat well and sparingly and follow the paleo diet guidelines. Some of the time, you can eat whatever you crave. And lots of it.

> Most of the time you need to eat well and sparingly and follow the paleo diet guidelines.

Rarely try a 100 percent/0 percent diet. You won't be able to do it for long, and your metabolism will down-regulate pretty fast. Those occasional splurges are what keep your metabolism humming along.

The anabolic burst

An anabolic burst is when you manipulate your diet and exercise in such a way that your body composition changes noticeably in a short period of time. It's a process of adding enough muscle and losing enough fat to be noticeable very quickly. This is the 100 percent/0 percent diet mentioned above. Used carefully and occasionally it can be a fun way to add muscle quickly.

How is this done? You start by eating very sparingly and 100 percent of the time according to the guidelines of the paleo diet for several weeks. At the same time, you exercise intensely. You then ease up on the exercise and go on an eating binge for up to five days. Your body will super-compensate. It will create amazing changes in a matter of a week or two.

After you've been training seriously for a while, you might consider experimenting with the anabolic burst. Before Thanksgiving, for example, train hard and maintain 100 percent paleo diet compliance. Then over a three or four-day Thanksgiving holiday, rest and eat as much as you can. See what your body does over the following week.

How do I know if my weight is good for me?

How much fat are you carrying? How much muscle? Is that proportion good or bad? This is where most authors explain the various options for testing your body composition. Pull out the calipers and pinch and measure and calculate. Or get an electrical impedance device such as a Tanita scale that will measure your percentage of body fat. Then you look at a chart that lists the percentage of body fat you should have, depending on your age and sex, and see how you rate. It's complicated, rife with opportunities for error, and it doesn't tell you anything about how much muscle you have.

> How much fat are you carrying? How much muscle? Is that proportion good or bad?

There's a better, simpler way. Just determine your ability to do chin-ups. Chin-ups enforce good body composition, a good balance between fat and muscle. This is a good test for both men and women. Men should be able to do at least three to six chin-ups, women, at least one to three. If you can't do even one chin-up, you're either carrying too much fat or not enough muscle, or likely both.

The skinny but fat phenomenon

Many women (and some men) look skinny, but have very little muscle mass. What they're made of is fat and bone instead of muscle and bone. Anyone who is thin, but unable to do any chin-ups is most likely an example of this phenomenon. Your weight may be low, but your body composition is off, and you need to add weight by adding muscle.

Remember that just being slim does not equal good body composition. After all, anorexics are thin, and they're certainly neither fit nor healthy. To be fit and healthy, you need a low percentage of body fat and a high percentage of muscle mass. This is why chin-ups are such a good indicator of body composition. To do them you need low body fat and enough muscle mass for your frame. Doing chin-ups is simple, straightforward, and less subject to error or interpretation than estimating percentage body fat in other ways.

> Just being slim does not equal good body composition.

Your body-mass index

Body-mass index (BMI) has become a popular measurement used to determine whether people are overweight. Our take, however, is that it's best to just ignore it. Why? Because it focuses on body *weight*, not body *composition*. Muscle weighs much more than fat. Athletes with a lot of muscle and a low percentage of body fat, for example, get BMI scores in the overweight category, while many fat people get a BMI score in the normal category. For our purposes, BMI scores are irrelevant.

Here's an example of how the BMI can be misleading. According to BMI, a 6 foot 2 inch tall powerlifter weighing 275 pounds is considered obese. But his body is heavily muscled with hardly any fat. And he can do 35 chin-ups. He is anything but obese. He is a huge, powerful athlete with great body composition.

When to eat?

When you eat is another critical factor. The right time to eat is after being active, not before. After you eat your body goes into digestion mode. Your muscles relax, and you become sleepy and less alert. Just think about trying to work after a big lunch. It's hard to stay awake. You yawn and down another cup of coffee, but it's still hard to get any productive work done.

Early evening is when you should eat your main meal. The day's activities are done, and after you eat you're relaxed and primed for sleep. It's interesting to note that our physiology also suggests that evening is the best time to eat the main meal of the day. Our metabolic rate in naturally lowest early in the morning and highest in the early evening. Our bodies are more ready for feeding in the evening than they were earlier in the day.

> The right time to eat is after being active, not before. After you eat your body goes into digestion mode. Your muscles relax, and you become sleepy and less alert.

Contrast how you feel after a large meal with how you feel when you're hungry. Like those Paleolithic hunters, when you're hungry, you're alert, active, and focused, often to the point of getting upset if your focus is disturbed. You're ready for action. In our evolutionary past, hunger was the signal to get going and hunt or forage for food. Even today we use the expression "he's hungry" to describe someone who wants something badly and is willing to work hard to get it.

The upshot of this is that during the day, when you're busy and active, you should keep yourself a bit hungry. Either fast or eat lightly. Then as you wind down around sunset or early in the evening, you can have a larger meal. Afterward, you'll be relaxed and ready for sleep.

What does it mean to eat lightly? It means snacking on a couple of hard-boiled eggs or some nuts and dried fruit. If you eat lunch, it can be something like a small chicken salad or a light soup. That's basically just a small amount of a food that our Paleolithic ancestors would recognize as food.

Of course, this goes against the current orthodoxy of continuous feeding, or eating four to six meals a day. But consider our history and evolution again. Human bodies have never before faced a continuous food supply. They are simply not able to handle it. Our bodies evolved to handle intermittent, unpredictable feedings. When faced with unlimited, continuous food, they don't know how to react or what to do. Is it any wonder that modern people have such a hard time staying lean and muscular?

Continuing research into the lifestyle of our hunter-gatherer ancestors supports eating less often every day. Again, Loren Cordain studying the pattern of daily meals among hundreds of hunter-gatherer groups found that the most common daily pattern was eating a single large meal in the evening. The next most common daily pattern was a large evening meal and a small breakfast of leftovers from the previous evening meal. These two patterns covered almost all the groups studied.

Now we come to the right time to eat those splurge meals, the 20 percent that don't need to be controlled. The special case regarding when to eat is after a hard workout of any type. That's when you need to eat a larger meal. At this point, and for a couple of hours afterward, your body is primed to assimilate nutrients faster and more efficiently. Taking advantage of this phenomenon will boost your fitness with almost no extra effort. It also makes sense from an evolutionary point of view. If you've just expended a lot of effort hunting or gathering, you need to put the fruits of your labor to work for your body as quickly as possible. So after every workout, even if it's in the morning, have something to eat.

> What does it mean to eat lightly? It means snacking on a couple of hard-boiled eggs or some nuts and dried fruit.

We may be modern humans, but we can't escape our evolutionary biology. This pattern of when to eat is ingrained in our biology. We can fight our bodies, but it's much easier, more effective, and healthier to work with them.

Supplements

Supplements can be of great help in our quest for higher levels of strength and conditioning. They work in two ways. First, they help us stay healthy. We can't train intensely if we're sick. Second, they can improve our training performance. Improved training leads to higher levels of strength and conditioning. Supplements that help you stay healthy are generally the nutrients your body needs to function properly. The best examples are water, electrolytes, vitamins, and minerals. If you become deficient in any of these, your body will just not work right.

But among nutritionists and medical professionals, there is a myth—the myth that a balanced diet will give us all of these basic nutrients in sufficient quantities. They tell us not only that we're wasting our money when we buy and take supplements, but also that taking high quantities of these basic nutrients could actually be harmful.

Don't believe it. First, these basic nutrients are not harmful. Even in very large doses, they are amazingly safe substances. Try to find a death caused by vitamin overdose. Yes, massive doses can cause side effects such as diarrhea or dry skin, but in all cases these effects quickly reverse when the dose is reduced.

Second, numerous studies measuring the levels of vitamins and minerals in large populations show clearly that almost everyone has some deficiency and many people are deficient in many nutrients.

For these reasons, you should make it a point to supplement your diet with these nutrients. It is good insurance to maintain your health. It gives you the ability to train intensely.

Supplements can also enhance training performance. There is quite a bit of overlap in supplements that improve health and those that enhance physical performance. After all, supplements that improve your health will improve your performance, and supplements that improve performance can also improve your health. An example of this is fish oil. Fish oil has been shown to improve health by fighting inflammation throughout the body and by reducing the incidence of heart arrhythmias. Both of these qualities also improve performance. A stronger heart will improve cardio training and reduced muscle inflammation will help your body build muscle and strength.

Use supplements. They will help your overall health. They will help you achieve your strength and conditioning goals. We discuss the supplements we use in the following paragraphs. We believe that this is a solid program that covers the basics. It has worked for us. We include a few less common supplements, too. We can definitely tell that when we're consistently taking our supplements. Our health and performance are noticeably better.

> Supplements that help you stay healthy are generally the nutrients your body needs to function properly. The best examples are water, electrolytes, vitamins, and minerals.

Water and salt.

Water and salt are not generally considered to be supplements, but if you're exercising intensely, they become critical. You need to make a special effort to consume enough water and salt.

We live in the high desert of California. The good news here is that the weather is sunny and warm fall, winter, and spring. The bad news is that the summers are brutally hot. As we've gotten older, we've noticed that it has become more difficult to exercise in the heat.

Having lived for decades just a few miles from Death Valley in a hot desert climate, we have experience with exercising outdoors in high heat. When it's hot, it's impossible to consume enough liquids while exercising intensely. Your rate of sweating is higher than the rate of absorption of liquid from your stomach. Dehydration is a given. That's why it's so important to rehydrate after every workout in the heat.

When you're exercising intensely outdoors, temperatures of 80 to 90° Fahrenheit qualify as hot and require close attention to hydration to prevent heat injury. When the temperatures climb up to 90 to 100° and you're exercising intensely, especially for more than one or two hours, it becomes very likely that you'll suffer dehydration and possibly heat injury. Temperatures of 100 to 110° or higher are dangerous. When the temperatures climb to these levels, prudence dictates that you work out indoors in an air conditioned venue.

It doesn't take much dehydration for you to feel it. Lose only three percent of your body weight, and your athletic performance will suffer and you'll feel exhausted and unwell. If you lose five percent or more of your body weight, it can quickly become a medical issue. Water loss of this magnitude leads to cramps, heat exhaustion, and even heatstroke. Dehydration is common when exercising hard in the heat. Even when he drinks two large water bottles (roughly one liter, or 2.2 pounds of water per bottle), Andy often loses five pounds (about three percent) or more of his 165 pound body weight during a two-hour bicycle ride during the summer. He feels heavy fatigue and lightheadedness. To rehydrate, he needs to drink at least five 16-ounce glasses of water.

With dehydration come electrolyte imbalances. For every pint of sweat you perspire, you lose electrolytes, primarily sodium. Loss of electrolytes can have a serious impact on the body, up to and including dangerous heart rhythm irregularities and brain issues such as loss of consciousness and even coma. Rehydrating by drinking lots of water, but neglecting to replace lost electrolytes can trigger such serious problems. This is sometimes referred to as water toxicity, but it's really lack of electrolytes in your blood plasma, that is, your blood becomes too dilute.

You must replace the water you're losing. And you must replace your electrolytes. You only need to be really concerned with sodium (salt, or sodium chloride) because the other electrolytes you lose are easily replaced by what you eat. Salt, which is critical if you're exercising in the heat, needs to be added to your diet. Low salt diets are simply incompatible with working out in the heat. Actually, they are incompatible with working out intensely, period. Even in cooler temperatures, you still sweat a lot. If you're on a low-salt diet, perhaps because of blood pressure issues, you must talk with a physician before exercising intensely or exercising in the heat. This is doubly critical because as we age, our sweating mechanisms become less efficient and less able to keep our body temperature under control. We sweat less, but our sweat is more concentrated.

One solution to rehydrating and replacing electrolytes is to drink one of the many modern sports drinks, almost all of which contain electrolytes, though the concentration tends to be relatively high. These may be optimum for athletes in their twenties, but they tend to be too concentrated for many older exercisers. Trying to rehydrate with sports drinks can result in bloating, nausea, diarrhea, and other uncomfortable side effects. Try one and see if it works for you. If it does, that's great. But if the sports drink doesn't work, we have another suggestion.

> If you're on a low-salt diet, perhaps because of blood pressure issues, you must talk with a physician before exercising intensely or exercising in the heat.

Try using an oral rehydration product like Pedialyte. Designed for infants who are dehydrated, this product is both very mild and very effective. That makes it also very effective for older athletes. (Obviously, as an adult you'll need to use more than suggested for infants.) Pedialyte is widely available without prescription in grocery and drug stores. The liquid form is great, but it also comes in strips that dissolve in the mouth that also work well with water and are very convenient. You can slip one of the tiny packs in a pocket.

How do you tell when you're sufficiently rehydrated? First, you should be passing urine. If you're not peeing, you're still dehydrated. Second, check the color of your urine. It should be a light, pastel yellow. If it's dark yellow, you still need to drink more. Also be aware that blood in the urine or urine that is a dark brown color (like the color of root beer) can be a sign of a serious medical problem like rhabdomyolysis, which can be brought on by hard efforts in high temperatures and dehydration and which can cause serious kidney damage. You need to seek medical attention right away! Rapid treatment with IV fluids and possibly dialysis can prevent permanent kidney damage.

We don't want to scare you here, but maintaining proper hydration and electrolyte balance while exercising intensely, especially in the heat, is absolutely vital to safety and enjoyment. Every year many people die or suffer serious injury because they don't pay attention to consuming enough water and salt. Don't be one of them.

Multivitamins and minerals.

When you take a good quality multivitamin and mineral every day, you can be sure that your body is getting sufficient vitamins and minerals to stay healthy. Don't be talked out of this by so-called experts that claim you can get all the necessary vitamins and minerals in sufficient quantities from your diet. Studies have shown that this just isn't true. And don't be dissuaded by anyone who tells you that they're too expensive. Being sick because of a deficiency is much more expensive. Bottom line? Take your vitamins and minerals.

Vitamin D.

Vitamin D, the "sunshine vitamin," is produced in your body when your skin is exposed to enough intense sunlight. Once thought necessary only for bone health and helping the body process calcium, vitamin D has been shown in recent studies to be important to your health in many other respects. Susceptibility to the flu and other respiratory infections, heart disease, stroke, heart failure, cancer, and premature death have all been linked to insufficient levels of vitamin D.

Thanks to reduced exposure to the sun in the winter, our increased use of sunscreens in the summer, and our modern indoor lifestyle, large portions of the U.S. population are deficient in vitamin D. For health purposes, you need to supplement with vitamin D. Taking 1,000 international units (IU) in the summer and 3,000 to 5,000 IU in the winter can ensure that your body's vitamin D levels remain adequate throughout the year. Vitamin D is reasonably cheap and can improve your overall health significantly.

Now a word about sunscreens. The so-called experts are constantly reminding us to generously apply sunscreen to avoid sunburn and skin cancer when we exercise outdoors and are exposed to the rays of the sun. This is bad advice. The sunscreen will clog your pores and inhibit your ability to sweat, which greatly increases the possibility of heat injury (heat exhaustion or heat stroke). Andy learned this lesson the hard way while riding a hilly century on a hot, sunny summer day. He applied sunscreen before the ride and noticed that he wasn't sweating when he was working hard uphill. His skin was getting hot to the touch. Soon he became nauseated and light-headed. He had to stop riding. This has never happened to him on any hard, hot ride when he wasn't using sunscreen. If you need to protect your skin from the sun, use clothing. There are now many hats and lightweight, mesh shirts and jerseys with long sleeves available that provide excellent sun protection.

Another alternative to using sunscreen is to exercise outdoors around dawn. Even in the height of summer, your exposure to the sun will be minimal if you're outside at this time. This is our preferred alternative because in the desert in the summer it's also the coolest time of day.

If you ride indoors, of course, you'll avoid any exposure at all. We think that this is pretty extreme, but it is an option.

Having made these recommendations, we urge you not to be paranoid about the sun. Some exposure is healthy, as it gives your body large amounts vitamin D along with other benefits. Only excessive exposure will age your skin and increase your chances of developing basal or squamous cell skin cancers. Fortunately, these skin cancers can be easily treated. Melanoma, the serious form of skin cancer, is not related to continuous heavy sun exposure, but rather intermittent intense sun exposure.[4] For example, in Australia, office workers have higher rates of melanoma than lifeguards. So if you avoid sunburns you reduce your chance of getting the severe form of skin cancer. Bottom line—get some sun, but don't overdo it. Use common sense.

Magnesium and calcium.

Magnesium and calcium are vital for the proper functioning of your heart and skeletal muscles. Magnesium is involved in proper relaxation, while calcium is involved in proper contraction. Magnesium has been shown to be vital for heart health. Since studies show that many people are not getting enough magnesium in their diets, it's important to make sure that you supplement with this mineral at a level of at least 400 milligrams (mg) a day. In addition to being a vital part of muscle contraction, calcium is also needed to build and maintain healthy bones. Since the paleo diet excludes milk products, it's a good idea to supplement with at least 800 mg a day.

A valuable side benefit of taking magnesium and calcium supplements is that the combination helps your muscles relax after intense exercise. The increased muscle tone from intense exercise can make muscles tight and "jumpy," which makes it hard to relax and sleep well. Supplementing with these minerals can help your muscles wind down and help you relax.

---

[4]J.M. Elwood, J.Jopson, (1997). Melanoma and sun exposure: an overview of published studies. In *J Cancer.* 73(2):198-203.

Fish oils.

It turns out that more important than the amount of fat in our diets is the *type of fat*. Some fats such, as trans fats and saturated fats, are bad for our health, while others, such as fish oils, are excellent. Fish oil has been studied extensively and found to be good for us on many levels. Two of the most notable benefits are that it fights inflammation and promotes heart health by preventing arrhythmias. Fish oils can improve our health and help us exercise more intensely.

Since most Americans don't eat much fish, especially the fattier fish like sardines and salmon, it's a good idea to take a fish oil supplement. Fish oil capsules are widely available and are the best supplement choice. They give you healthy fish oils without the nasty taste of cod liver oil, which was very popular in the past. Cod liver oil is a good source of fish oils, but most people won't use it consistently because of the bad taste. Six grams a day is enough to get the benefits of this supplement.

> Fish oil has been studied extensively and found to be good for us on many levels. Two of the most notable benefits are that it fights inflammation and promotes heart health by preventing arrhythmias.

Protein and creatine.

One of the best supplements for anyone who exercises intensely is the protein shake. Consumed right after exercise, when your body's refueling and repair mechanisms are working in overdrive, a good protein shake will do more to enhance your physical performance than any other supplement. Refueling during this window of opportunity that lasts from when you stop exercising to two or three hours later is thus critically important. Fast acting whey protein in your shake will make the protein quickly available to your muscles to aid in their rebuilding progress. Your body will have one of the critical building blocks for muscles repair. Adding creatine to your shake will help your muscles cells absorb water and rehydrate. This makes the muscle cells work more efficiently by making them stronger.

Since the paleo diet excludes milk, we've come up with a simple combo that's a tasty alternative to a protein shake using milk. Combine four ounces of unsweetened apple sauce with four ounces of water and then add a scoop of whey protein powder, which is the best type because it's assimilated into the body the fastest. Then add one teaspoon (five grams) of creatine monohydrate, which is available as a powder and is very effective in increasing muscular strength. You can eat it plain (with a spoon) or add nuts and whole or sliced fruit to make it tastier. We like to add walnuts and fruit like bananas, apples, strawberries, raspberries, blueberries, or raisins.

> Consumed right after exercise, when your body's refueling and repair mechanisms are working in overdrive, a good protein shake will do more to enhance your physical performance than any other supplement.

This shake is plenty for after a strength or muscular endurance session and any bike ride of two hours or less. However, if we're back from a three to five-hour ride, we need more, so we'll add a nutrition bar or two if the ride was especially brutal. Alternatively, a peanut butter and jelly sandwich or some brownies can be good choices.

Beta-alanine.

Beta-alanine is an amino acid that works to increase the carnosine levels in your muscles. Carnosine, a dipeptide of the amino acids beta-alanine and histidine, is highly concentrated in muscles. Greater carnosine levels result in muscles that are stronger and have greater endurance. Used together, creatine and beta-alanine can lead to noticeable increases in strength and muscular endurance.[5]

Studies have shown that supplementing with 1.5 to 3.0 grams of beta-alanine a day increases the concentration of carnosine in the muscles of both young adults and older men and women (ages 55 to 92). More importantly, these studies also showed that people receiving beta-alanine supplementation were able to exercise more intensely before becoming fatigued.[6] Reduced feelings of fatigue while exercising make consistently engaging in intense exercise easier.

Coenzyme Q (COQ).

This is vital to fuel the mitochondria in all your cells, including your muscle cells. Mitochondria are the powerhouses of your cells that convert chemicals from your food into energy that powers cell functions. In the mitochondria, COQ aids in the conversion of ATP (Adenosine-triphosphate, an energy storage chemical) into energy. It's especially vital to a healthy heart. Heart muscle is dense with mitochondria, and sufficient COQ maximizes the efficiency of the heart. Having sufficient COQ to power the mitochondria in your heart is especially vital if you take any statin drug for high cholesterol. Statin drugs block the production of COQ in the liver (where it's normally produced), resulting in deficiency. Muscle mitochondria lacking COQ cause the muscles to become weak and sore. This is the basis of the side effect of muscle weakness and soreness when taking statins. The heart muscle can also become weak from a lack of COQ.

---

[5] J. J. Wilson, G. J. Wilson, et al. (2010) Beta-alanine supplementation improves aerobic and anaerobic indices of performance. *Strength and Cond J.* 32(1):71-78.

[6] J.R. Hoffman, et al. (2008) Short-duration beta-alanine supplementation increases training volume and reduces subjective feelings of fatigue in college football players. *Nutr Res.* 28:31-35.

If you're taking statins, therefore, be sure to supplement with coenzyme Q. You should take at least 100 to 200 mg a day. Even if you're not on a statin drug, taking supplemental COQ is good for your heart and every other muscle in your body. Fifty to 100 mg a day is appropriate, especially if you're stressing it by doing intense exercise.

ZMAT (men only) .

A supplement composed of zinc and magnesium along with the herb *terribilis*, ZMAT has been shown to support natural testosterone production in your body. The more testosterone your body has, the greater strength and conditioning gains you'll make from your training efforts. ZMAT is a viable alternative to using steroids. Its effect is not nearly as dramatic, but it does work. Andy feels (and actually is) stronger and recovers from workouts faster when he uses it.

About steroids

First, a reality check. Steroids work. Training plus steroids will make you stronger, faster, more muscular, leaner, etc., than the same training without steroids. Also, when they're used properly, steroids are generally safe. Think about it. Steroids are used to treat people with many different ailments including serious, life-threatening diseases like AIDS. If they're safe for sick people, they are certainly safe for use by healthy people. It's *steroid abuse* that is not safe. Keep in mind, however, that the abuse of any drug can be dangerous. The medical community has lost credibility among athletes because of the continuing claims of physicians that steroids don't work and are dangerous. Anyone who has experience with these drugs knows that this just isn't true.

A reality check. Steroids work. Training plus steroids will make you stronger, faster, more muscular, leaner, etc., than the same training without steroids. Also, when they're used properly, steroids are generally safe.

That said, before you decide whether or not to use steroids, consider some other ramifications. First, steroids are now banned in almost all sports and there are significant penalties for getting caught cheating. Also, consider the abuse potential and the dangers, such as non-sterile needle infections and, especially if you use black market drugs, possible contamination or fake drugs. And don't forget that if you don't have a doctor's prescription, the possession of steroids is a serious drug offense that could land you in jail for a long stretch.

It may be tempting to use steroids to push your strength and conditioning to the highest levels, but the risks involved are great. Use other supplements, but think about it long and hard before you start down the path of steroid use. We've made the decision to not use steroids and recommend that you make the same decision.

Final words about supplements

Remember that supplements are *supplemental to a good paleo diet*, not a substitute for nutrition. Generally speaking, the best time to take most supplements is with meals. Supplements can not only play a part in keeping you in good health, but they can also help you reach your strength and conditioning goals. Keep your supplement program simple, however, and focus on those that have been shown to be effective in maintaining health and improving performance.

8 What About Flexibility?

Flexibility is a Goldilocks phenomenon. You want enough, but not too much. You want to have a normal range of motion. Why? Because a normal range of motion lets your body work like it should, which maximizes the efficiency of your movement and prevents injury. What's a normal range of motion? There are elaborate tests, but really it's pretty simple. You should be able to (1) bend over forward and touch your toes, (2) go down into a full squat, and (3) clasp your hands behind your back.

Left: You should be able to touch your toes.

Center: You should be able to drop into a full squat.

Right: And you should be able to clasp your hands behind your back.

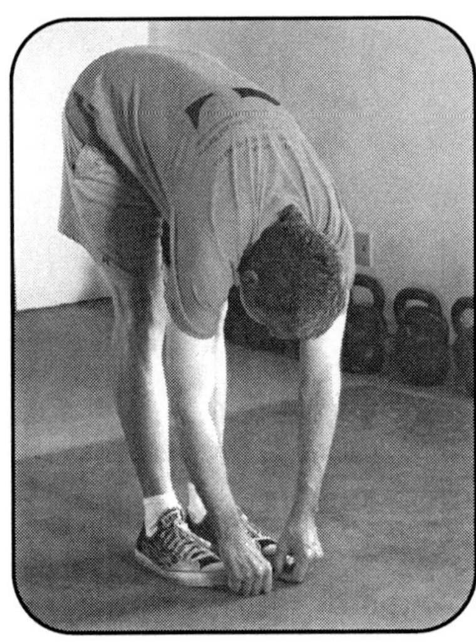
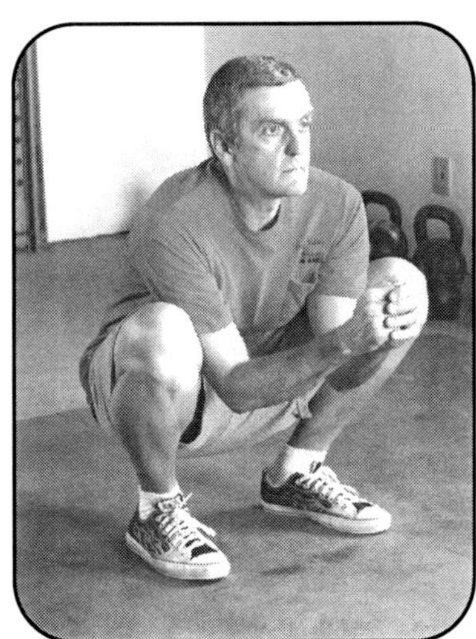
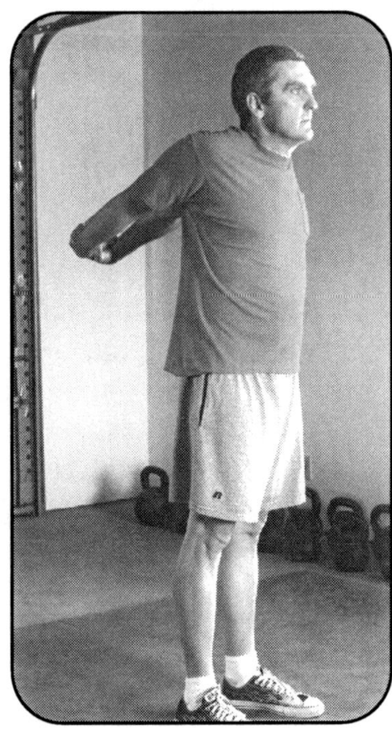

Notice that what is commonly referred to as flexibility has two components. The first is muscle tightness. The second is joint mobility.

Before we talk about how to stretch and how to improve joint mobility, we need to make a very important point. To stay functionally flexible, you don't really need to stretch or do joint mobility work. If you do your strength and kettlebell exercises with a full range of motion, this alone will maintain a functional level of flexibility. Additionally, if you perform ballistic kettlebell exercises, such as snatching and/or cleaning and jerking, those are excellent for joint health. The repetitive impact loads that these exercises put on your joints strengthen them and keep them healthy. Joints subject to the heavy but brief impact that kettlebells impose adapt and become stronger and better able to handle the normal stresses of walking, running, jumping, and lifting. And joints that are exercised in this way are also relatively free of osteoarthritis in old age, as compared to joints that aren't exercised like this.

> If you do your strength and kettlebell exercises with a full range of motion, this alone will maintain a functional level of flexibility.

Keeping your joints mobile and your muscles limber will give you the flexibility you need to do what you want to do. So, if needed, do some joint mobility exercises and/or a little stretching every day. Consistency (a little every day) is much better than doing a lot occasionally, like that once-a-week yoga class. Also, don't go overboard and think you need the flexibility of a pretzel. For almost everyone, achieving and maintaining a normal range of motion should be the goal of flexibility work.

Stretching

Tight muscles can prevent a full range of motion. When you use various techniques to relax your muscles, you can restore that range of motion. But note that once you have a full range of motion, stretching farther becomes counterproductive. Lax muscles don't stabilize joints, and unstable joints can invite injury.

That said, if you have issues with tight muscles and want to do more, here are some suggestions. There are several ways to stretch, including ballistic stretching and static, yoga-like, slow stretching. Much more effective than these types of stretching is the tense-release method. Simply move into a position that slightly stretches a muscle you want to stretch and then tense it. After tensing it, release the tension. You will feel the muscle lengthen. Repeat this until you no longer feel the muscle lengthen during the release. It helps if you inhale and hold your breath while tensing and then exhale as you relax your muscles.

> Tight muscles can prevent a full range of motion.

Let's use your hamstrings as an example. To stretch your hamstrings, bend over like you're going to touch your toes. Then inhale and tighten up your hamstrings. Your fingers will come up slightly. Now exhale and release the tension. As your hamstrings lengthen, you'll be reaching further down toward your toes. Repeat this tense-release cycle, matching it with your breathing until you touch your toes or are no longer experiencing further muscle lengthening.

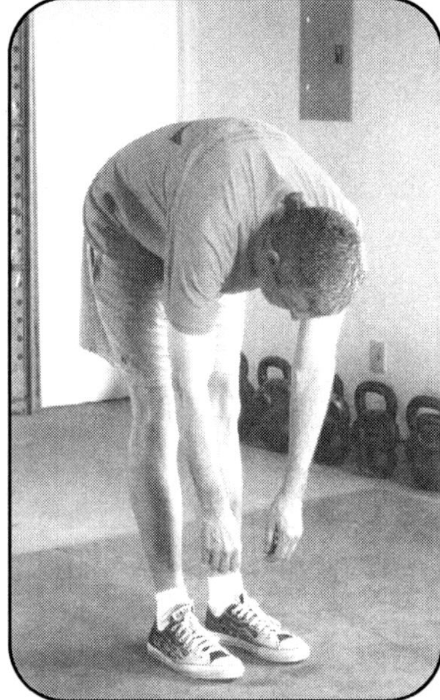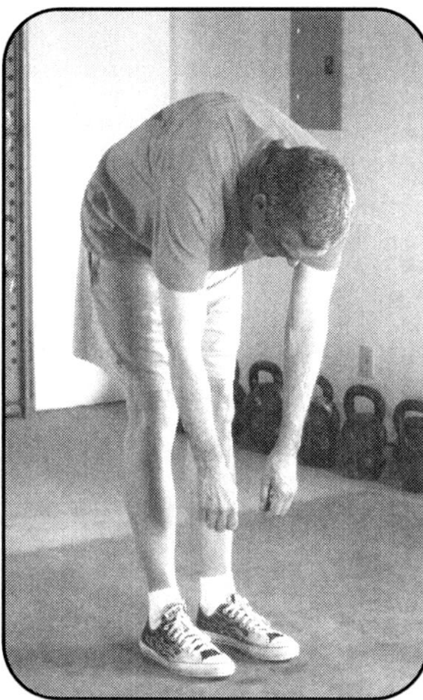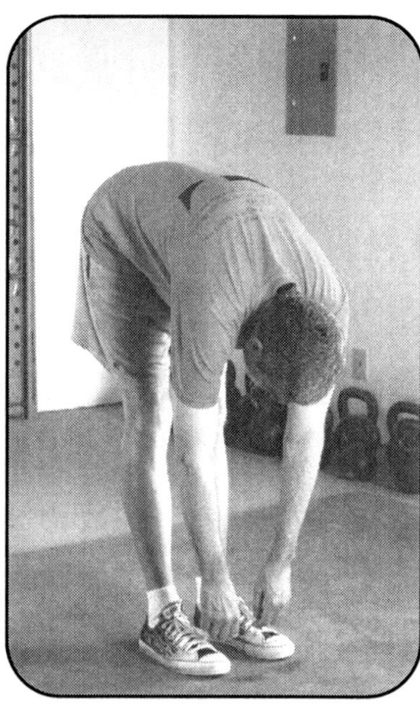

Tense-release hamstring stretch. Note how the fingers come up while tensing and then drop down into a deeper stretch when the tension is released.

Another example. You want to be able to comfortably squat deeper. Go down into a squat and tighten up the muscles in your lower body as you inhale. You'll come up slightly as you tense. Now exhale and relax. You'll find yourself naturally sinking into a deeper squat. Repeat as needed to reach the level you want. This tense-release method of stretching can increase your range of motion and loosen up tight muscles. Use it when you need to for these purposes.

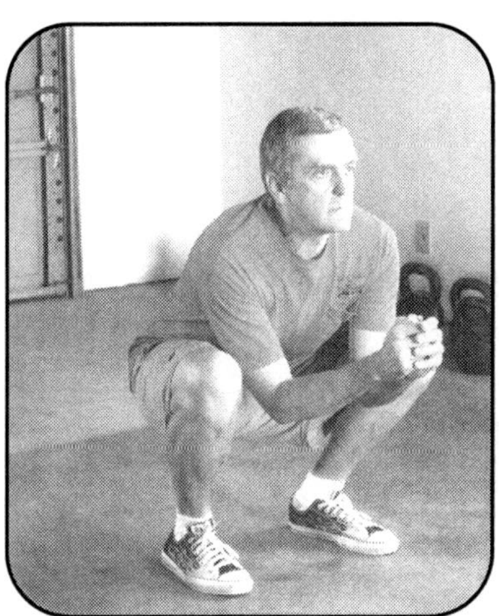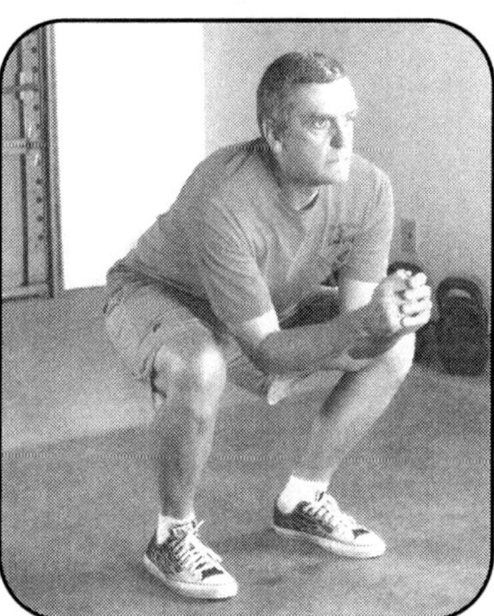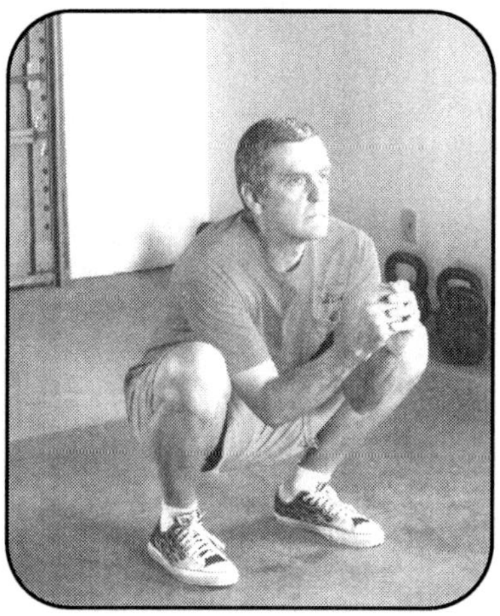

Tense-release squat stretch. Note how the body comes up while tensing and then drops down into a deeper squat when the tension is released.

Joint mobility

Joint mobility is the ability of the joints to move smoothly through a full range of motion. As we all get older, we really need to maintain joint mobility. We need to make a point of moving our joints through a full range of motion every day. If you have issues with stiff joints you can exercise to restore their mobility. How do you do that? In a word, *motion*. Moving your joints through their full range of motion keeps the joints mobile and lubricated.

Start with your toes. Clench and release them. Then move your ankles in circles, first clockwise, then counter-clockwise. Move up to your knees. Bend them slightly, put your hands on them, and move them in circles in both directions. Get your hips moving by circling them like you're using a hula hoop. Body weight squats can finish up your joint mobility work for your lower body.

> As we all get older, we really need to maintain joint mobility. We need to make a point of moving our joints through a full range of motion every day.

Follow the same process for your upper body. Start by clenching and unclenching your fingers. Then move on to wrist circles, elbow circles, and shoulder circles, working them to make the biggest circles you can.

Loosen up your spine by bending forward and backward in alternate motions. Many people have tight necks. Mobilize your neck by first bending your head forward and backward, then from side to side, and finally rotate from side to side.

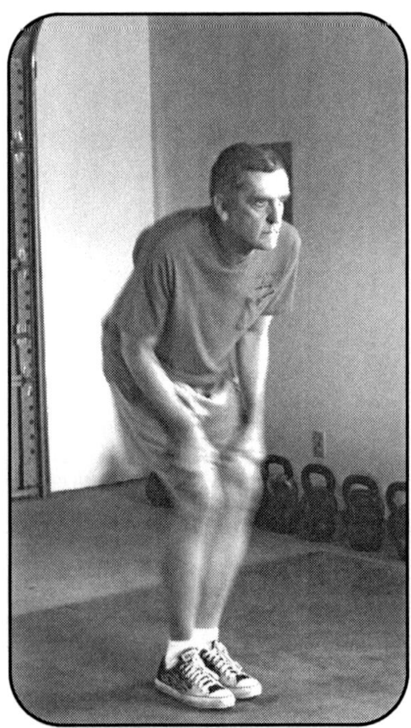

Joint mobility - knee circles.

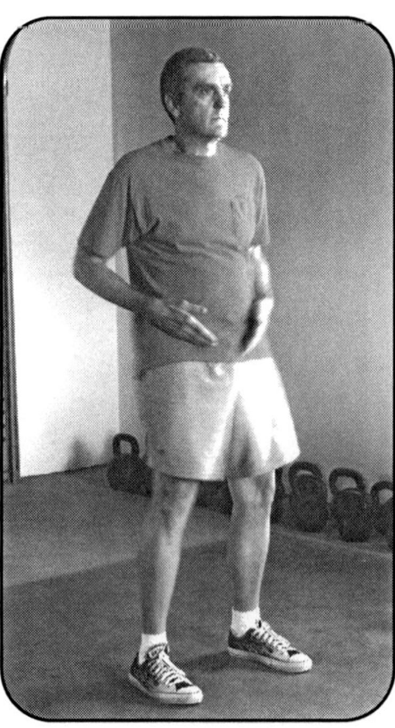

Joint mobility - hip circles.

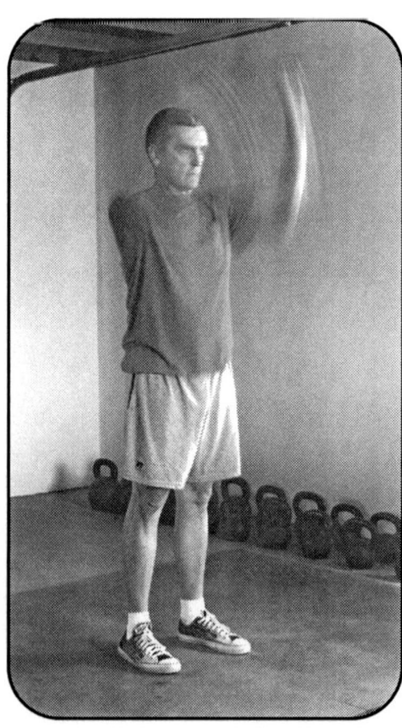

Joint mobility - arm circles.

Moving your joints every day will keep them lubricated and mobile. A good rule of thumb is to do the same number of reps as your age. So if you're 50 you do 50 repetitions (25 clockwise plus 25 counterclockwise) of each joint mobility exercise. Of course, you should always start out easy with only a few repetitions and work up over time to your age number.

Warming up before intense exercise

A topic closely related to flexibility is warming up before intense exercise. Nowadays, the conventional wisdom is that you need to do extensive warm-ups. You need to raise the temperature of your entire body and muscles until you're sweating, and then you need to work the specific movement to get your muscles primed. For example, if you followed this advice, you would jog on a treadmill for a few minutes and then lift a few sets of the Sumo deadlift using light weights before going on to heavier working weights.

> Many exercise "experts" and some coaches and trainers who should know better still advocate stretching as part of a warm-up. We believe that this is a truly counterproductive practice.

In addition, many exercise "experts" and some coaches and trainers who should know better still advocate stretching as part of a warm-up. We believe that this is a truly counterproductive practice that relaxes muscles that actually need to be tight to be primed for action. Remember that tension equals strength, whereas stretching equals relaxation. Never, ever stretch before exercise as part of a warm-up. You can include some stretching as part of a cool-down as a way to relax and wind down from exercise, but it should not be part of your warm-up.

When people follow the conventional warm-up wisdom to do extensive warm-ups, what often happens is that they spend a lot more time warming up than actually doing any intense exercise.

We believe that most of this time spent warming up is simply wasted time. We started thinking about this while watching the rabbits on our property. When we walk around the land, the rabbits nearby will freeze, usually under a creosote bush. As we approach them, we can see that their muscles are so tense that they're quivering. When we get too close, the bunnies bolt. They go from a complete stop with tensed muscles to a full run in a flash. We've never seen them warming up with some jumping jacks and bodyweight squats before they start running. They just go. Their muscles evolved for this kind of effort. Rabbits that couldn't run fast in an instant were culled from the gene pool. They were eaten.

Applying this observation to humans, there are two points to make. First, rabbit muscles are functionally the same as human muscles. They work in the same manner and should thus be capable of similar efforts. Second, from an evolutionary perspective, early humans needed the same abilities as rabbits. On the African savannah, when a lion spotted you, you didn't have time to warm up. You had to run for your life *right now* or risk being removed from the gene pool.

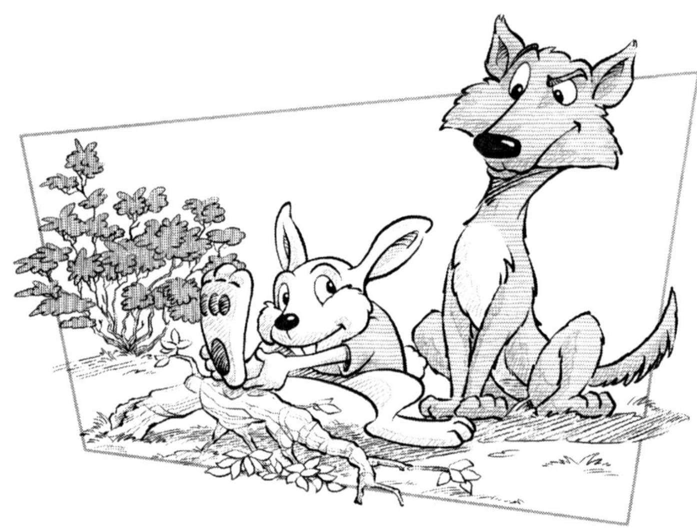

Just a sec…I need to stretch my hamstrings.

What does this tell us? Warm-ups may make exercise more psychologically comfortable, but there is no real physical reason to do them. They are just not needed. As you start to train without warm-ups, your body and mind will quickly adapt. You'll have more time for productive intense efforts.

Having made our case against warm-ups, the reality is that most of you will continue with the practice. In that case, let us encourage you to keep them short. We suggest a few minutes of joint mobility work followed by a set of 10 to 20 bodyweight squats and a set of 5 to 10 push-ups.

Cooling down after exercise

As with warm-ups, extensive cool-downs are simply not necessary after exercise. Just walk or bike easily, keeping your muscles moving for a few minutes. Once your breathing and heart rate settle down, you're done.

If you need to stretch to loosen up tight muscles, this is a good time to do that. There's no need for anything more extensive or complicated.

9
Good Equipment Is a Necessity

Successful strength and conditioning training requires equipment. Buy your own equipment and keep it handy in your garage or basement or spare room (or living room, where for many years Andy kept his bicycle and trainer). The number one rule of buying training equipment is to buy the best you can. Good equipment makes training easier and more fun. Better equipment will make you a better athlete. So don't skimp. You don't need the gold-plated, top-of-the-line, but you do need top quality.

Some of the equipment you need is available in gyms, although we've observed that most gyms don't actually have much equipment that's really useful except barbells and dumbbells. And if you want to use the gym's equipment, of course, you have to get there and back and you have to compete with other patrons. Not to mention that many of us in the older generation don't much like the current gym scene with its pounding music and all those brightly, tightly clad young people doing more socializing than exercising. Gyms today are designed for a younger demographic. They can be intimidating, embarrassing, irritating, and frustrating venues for those of us who want to accomplish any serious physical work. And consider your finances, too—you can buy a lot of exercise equipment for the cost of a yearly gym membership.

> The number one rule of buying training equipment is to buy the best you can. Good equipment makes training easier and more fun.

Exercising at home can definitely be preferable. Let's start with the basic equipment that you'll need to effectively train at home.

Shoes

Good shoes are vital. Of course you'll need different shoes for different purposes.

For lifting weights or kettlebells, *avoid* any sports shoe with padding, arch supports, or shock-absorbing gel. These kinds of shoes will throw off your balance and make it more difficult to lift weights because your feet will not be in solid contact with the ground. To safely and strongly lift weights you need to be properly balanced and be able to push firmly against the ground with your feet. Instead, lift barefoot or as close to barefoot as you can. Ballet or deadlift slippers, wrestling shoes, or sneakers such as Chuck Taylors with flat rubber soles and no padding are all good choices. The new Vibram Five Finger shoes are currently popular and are also excellent for lifting. Working out in your socks is not a good idea because socks tend to be slippery on many surfaces. Slipping while under weights can definitely be dangerous.

For bicycling, you need to acquire stiff-soled bicycling shoes with cleats that attach the shoes to the pedals. You will be amazed how much more comfortable and efficient pedaling will be.

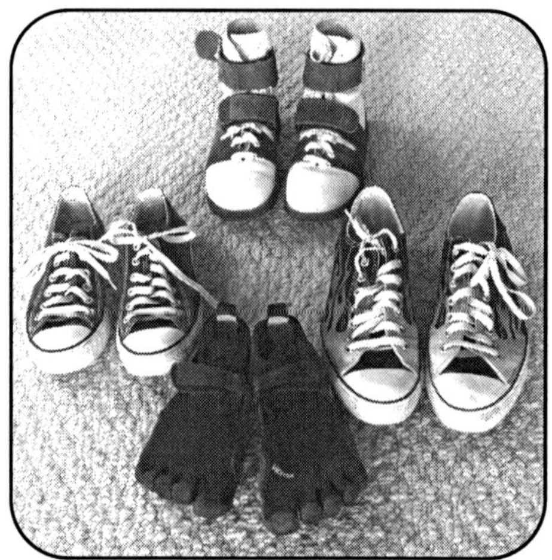

Shoes for weightlifting or kettlebell lifting – flat soles and no padding.

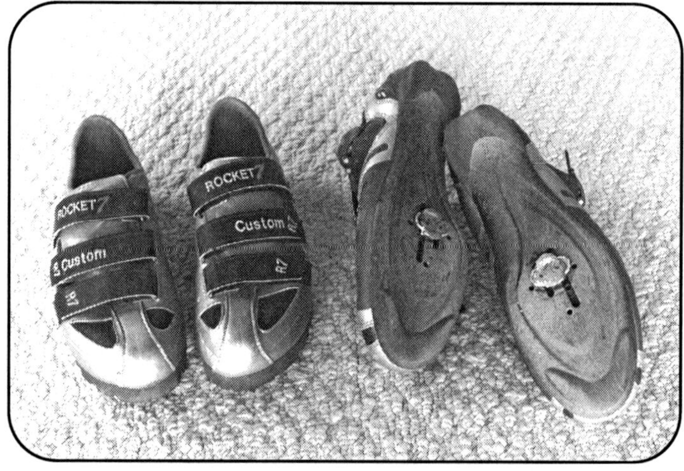

Shoes for bicycling – stiff soles with pedal cleats.

Straps, chalk, wrist bands

You need a strong grip to lift weights. As you lift heavier and heavier weights, your grip will strengthen naturally . . . unless you use lifting straps. Don't use straps. They'll help a little in the short run, but in the long term, they will hinder your strength development.

Do use chalk on your hands. It can prevent slippage due to sweaty hands, which will help you lift up to your ability.

Padded wrist sweatbands can help protect your wrists when you're doing kettlebell presses, snatches, and/or clean and jerks. Bruised wrists are painful, and some added protection can make kettlebell lifting much more pleasant.

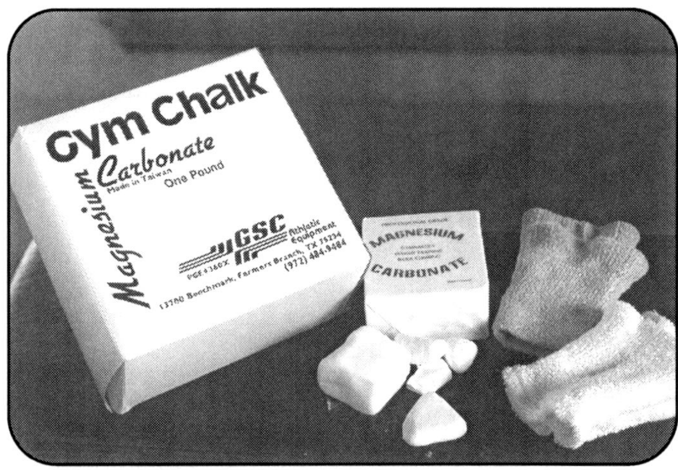

Approved aids for weightlifting or kettlebell lifting.

Lifting belts

Properly used when you are lifting very heavy weights, a real lifting belt can be an important safety accessory. "Very heavy" means you're lifting close to the maximum weight that you're capable of lifting. Which means you're competing in powerlifting. If this is what you're doing, then a thick, tight belt like those sold by Inzer is a wise investment.

For everyone else, however, a lifting belt is just a fashion accessory. The belt can provide a false sense of security and will most likely just prevent your back from getting stronger instead of preventing injury.

Generally speaking, just say no to fashion belts and lift without artificial support.

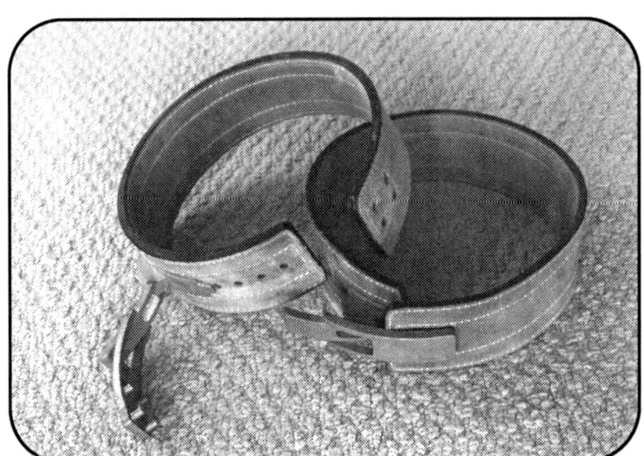

"Real" weightlifting belts – note the thick leather construction and heavy duty metal closures. Use this when lifting truly heavy weights.

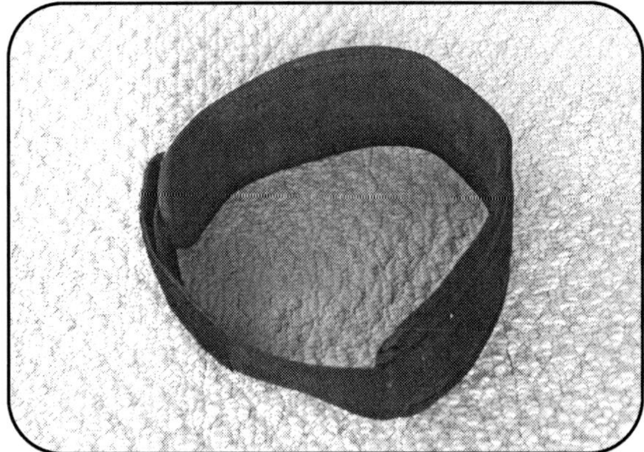

"Fashion" weightlifting belt – thin nylon with Velcro to hold it in place. No excuse to ever use this kind of belt.

Barbell and weight plates

If you're going to lift weights, you're going to need a barbell bar and weight plates. Buy a high quality Olympic barbell with rotating collars. These are not expensive and will last a lifetime, so buy the best. A standard Olympic bar will weigh 45 pounds. To deadlift properly, you'll need two 45-pound iron plates (to put the bar at the correct height). If 135 pounds is too much for you, five kilogram (11 pound) rubber bumper plates that are the same diameter as 45 pound iron plates are available. Almost everyone can deadlift 67 pounds, but if that's too heavy, you can start by deadlifting kettlebells.

Depending on your level of strength, you will also need an assortment of smaller iron weight plates. Start with pairs of plates weighing 1.25 pounds, 2.5 pounds, 5 pounds, 10 pounds, and 25 pounds. Then add more as needed. Weight plates are cheap and will last for your lifetime so get enough so that you can move up and down in weight in small percentage increments as well as challenge yourself.

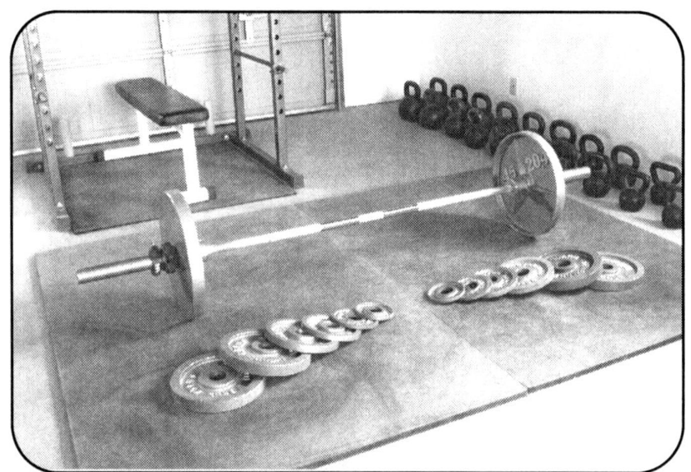

Olympic barbell with iron plates.

Kettlebells

High quality, Russian-design, cast-iron kettlebells with thick handles are a bit more expensive than cheaper models, but go ahead and buy them. You can find them at www.dragondoor.com. These bells are almost indestructible and will last for your lifetime and beyond.

Don't buy cheap knock-off kettlebells with thin handles made of rubber, plastic, or steel. These have bad balance and proportions. Kettlebell exercises were developed using the Russian design. Using kettlebells with

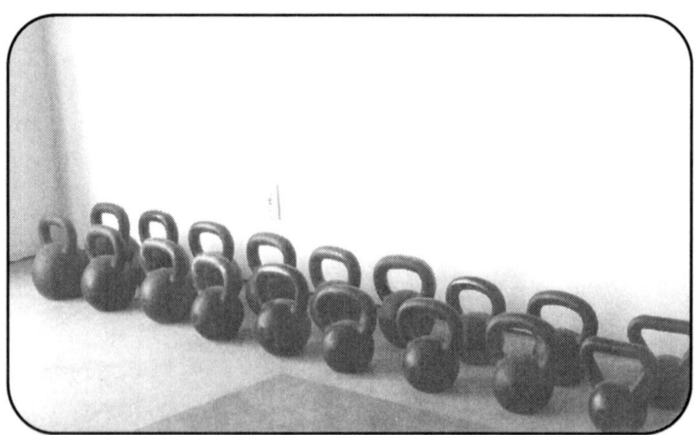

Kettlebells. This is a complete set. You can start with one or two.

the proper balance and proportions makes learning and doing the exercises much easier and safer.

Start with one size kettlebell and buy more as you progress in your training.

Lifting platform

A lifting platform is simply a flat, solid platform that you can stand on while lifting barbells and kettlebells. It has a non-slip surface to enhance lifting safety and is thick enough to protect the floor underneath. Whether you lift weights on the cement floor in your garage or a wood or tile floor in your house, a lifting platform will protect it from being damaged by iron weights being dropped on it. This also enhances safety; if you don't have to worry about damaging your floor, you won't have any hesitation in dropping the weight if a lift goes bad.

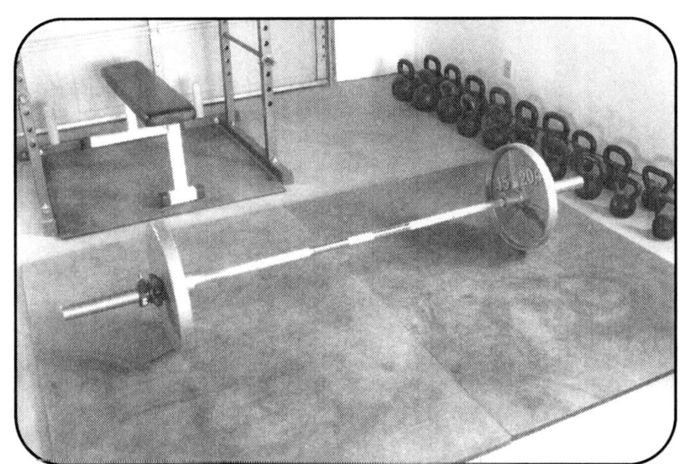

A simple but excellent lifting platform – two 4 foot by 6 foot dense rubber horse stall mats laid side to side.

A lifting platform can be something like two sheets of plywood with a non-slip surface applied or an eight-foot by eight-foot area of rubber floor tiles. The best option we've come across is to go to a local feed store and buy two horse stall mats. These mats are four feet by six feet in size and made of three-quarter-inch thick, dense rubber. Two of these mats laid next to each other form a large and high quality lifting platform. And the best part, they only cost about $40 each (2008 prices).

Chin-up bar

This is a solid bar from which you can do chin-ups. Ideally, it will be high enough so that you can hang straight and your feet don't touch the floor, but as long as it's high enough that your knees don't touch the floor, it'll work. The best choice is a free standing chinning bar or a power cage designed for powerlifting training that includes a chinning bar. These are readily available and not that expensive. High quality models start at around $200 (2012 prices). Alternatively,

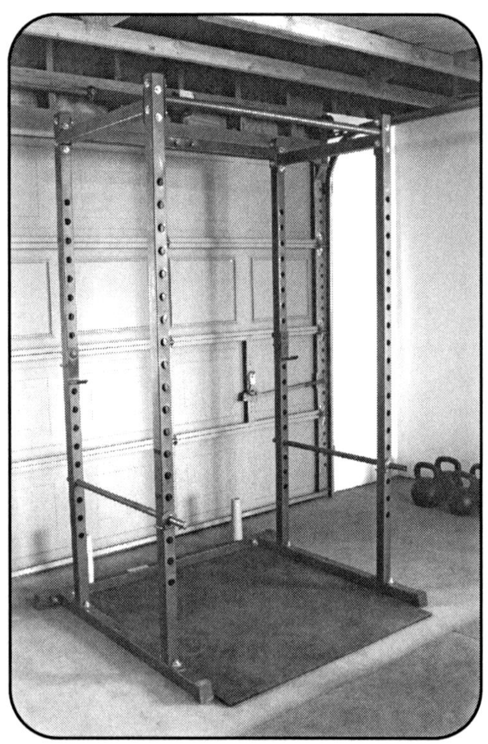

A solid chinning bar is part of
a powerlifting cage.

you can build a chinning bar from steel pipe that you can attach to the rafters in your garage or basement. Avoid the cheap chinning bars that attach to door frames. They aren't sturdy enough to safely support most people. Having one give way while you're doing a chin-up can result in a nasty and totally unnecessary injury.

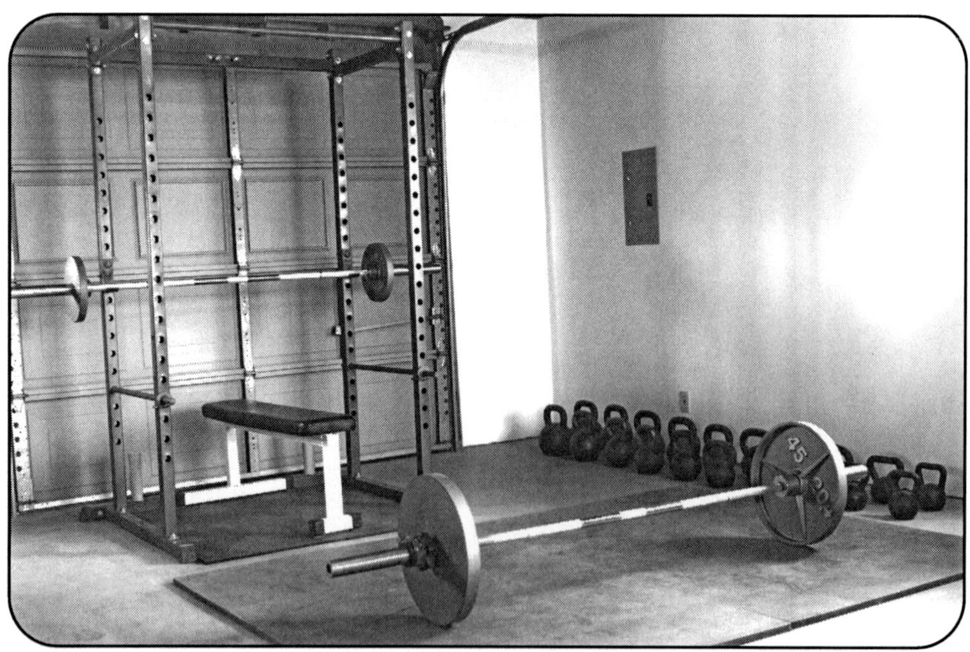

A complete home gym with everything needed for you to build strength and become lean and muscular – it easily fits in a garage.

High-quality road or mountain bike

A good bicycle is one of the most expensive items you'll need. If you're going to ride on paved roads, you'll need a high-quality, racing-style, road bike. If you're going to ride on dirt roads, you'll need a high-end, full-suspension, mountain bike. Well, you don't actually "need" a high-quality road or full-suspension mountain bike, but you'll be working more efficiently and comfortably if you choose one. You'll also enjoy riding a lot more if you go ahead and invest in one. And make no mistake—enjoying yourself every time you go out to ride is hugely important. It'll make staying consistent with your cardio training fun and easy instead of being a chore. And

that means you'll be able to improve and maintain that cardio conditioning and cardio health years into the future.

Expect to spend at least $1,500 to $3,000 (2012 prices). Bite the bullet. Buy the best you can afford. The improved ride quality makes riding more comfortable and much more fun. As you get in better condition and ride more, you'll appreciate how a good bike makes bicycling better.

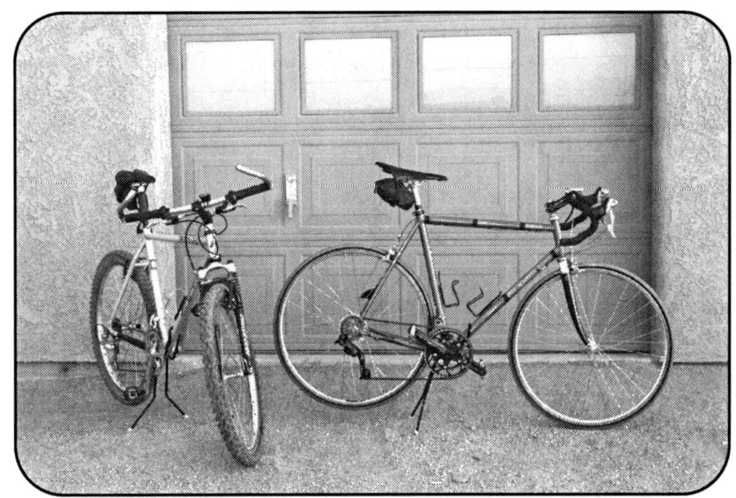

A quality road or mountain bike is invaluable for building cardio fitness.

Power meter

You'll spend another $500 to $1,500 (or more) for this electronic device, but you must choose one of the many models now available. There is no option. To truly effectively measure and train to increase your cardio fitness using a bicycle, you need a power meter.

Get a model that you can download to a PC or Mac. When you download the data and analyze it using software, you'll get the most information and benefits from using the power meter.

Andy has experience with several different brands of power meters. Some are easy to use, some more difficult. Some have loads of features that most of you won't use, and with others, you need more features. His opinion is that at the current time (2012) the CycleOps Power Tap is the best choice for people who are serious about their cardio training. It has all the features needed, is easy to use, and is reliable. There are several models available, including modestly priced ones in the $500 to $1,000 range. There are other meters that are also good, but considering price and performance, the Power Tap comes out on top.

Almost all power meters now come with analysis software, most of which is very good. Learn how to use it. Be sure that your software includes TSS score calculation. Right now, the best third-party software is Training Peak's software, but for most of us who aren't professional cyclists, this is overkill because it has loads of features that average athletes don't need. Focus on learning how to use that software that comes with your power meter and leave the complicated third party software to the pros.

To learn how to use your power meter and software to their full capabilities, get a copy of *Training and Racing with a Power Meter* by Hunter Allen and Andrew Coggan, Ph.D. This excellent book is currently the best available on this topic.

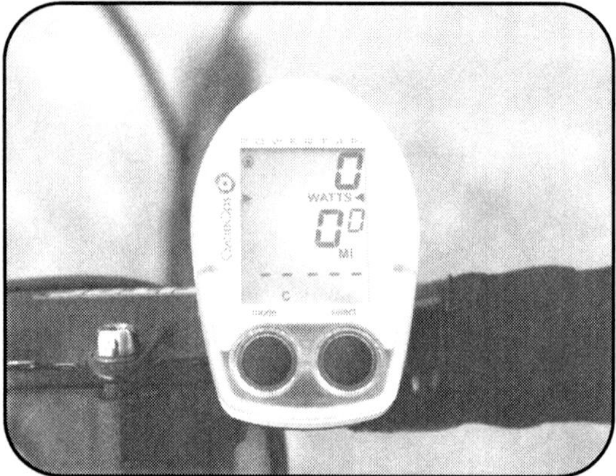

Power meter – this is the handlebar mounted computer head unit.

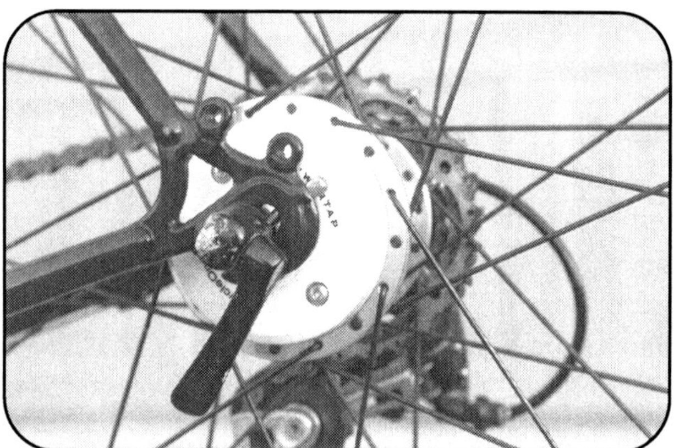

Power meter – this is the hub that contains the strain gauges that collect the power data.

Heart rate monitor

Good news here. Almost all power meters now include a heart rate monitor. The chest strap is included. Just strap it on, and the power meter will display and record your heart rate.

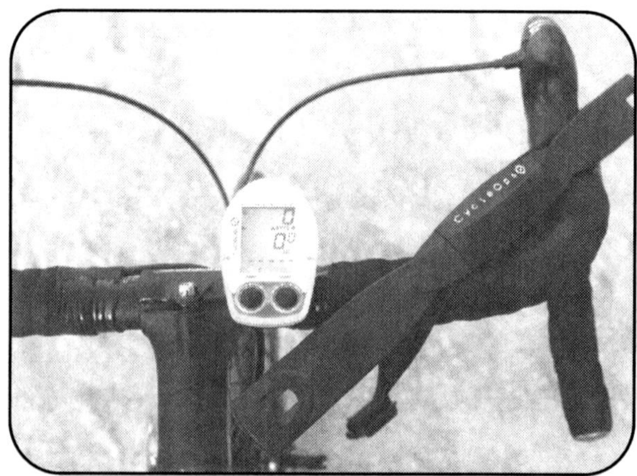

A heart rate monitor is built into most power meters – and the chest strap is included.

Indoor bicycle trainer

Bicycling is most fun when done outdoors, but with an indoor trainer you can train on your bike when you aren't able or don't want to ride outside, as in the winter, when it's too cold and/or too dark to ride outdoors, or if you live in a big city where it's impractical to ride on the busy streets. Or maybe you're just busy and want to do your cardio training in the most efficient way possible. An indoor trainer lets you do it.

Almost all power meters measure power via drive train torque, which means they work just as well on a trainer as they do on the road. The CycleOps Power Tap is an example of a power meter that works just as well on a trainer as on the road or trail.

Whenever you train indoors—in a garage, in the basement, or in any room inside your house—you'll also need a fan. Riding while stationary will result in producing buckets of sweat. A fan can make your exercise much more comfortable. Towels are also a must, one on the handlebars to wipe your head and neck, and maybe a couple on the floor to sop up flying sweat (required if you're training in your living room).

An indoor trainer can be more time efficient than riding outdoors. You get on, warm up for 5 to 10 minutes, complete your intervals, cool down for 5 minutes and get off. *Done*. It's done, but it's less fun than riding outdoors.

Buy a high-quality trainer, which will be smoother and more comfortable, making it easier to use and more likely to be used. The two most important features to look for are magnetic drive-fluid resistance and a large flywheel. Magnetic drive-fluid resistance is resistance provided by a fan rotating in an enclosed fluid (usually some type of oil) chamber. This arrangement provides smoothly increasing resistance and is quiet. You want a magnetic drive because the oil is in a sealed container. Shaft drives tend to leak oil from around the shaft seal, which can create

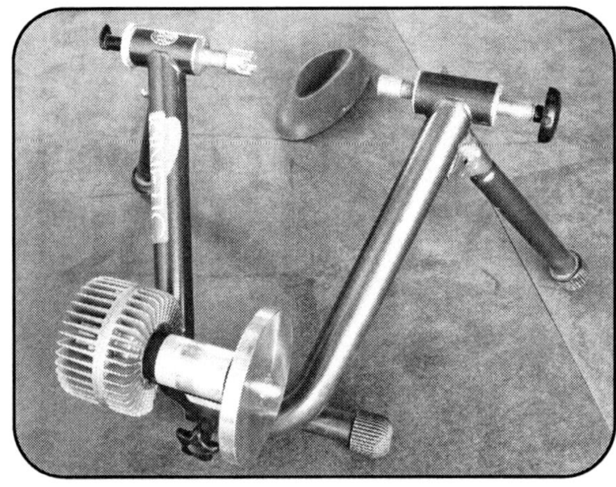

A quality bike trainer with a front wheel riser that's used to keep the bike level.

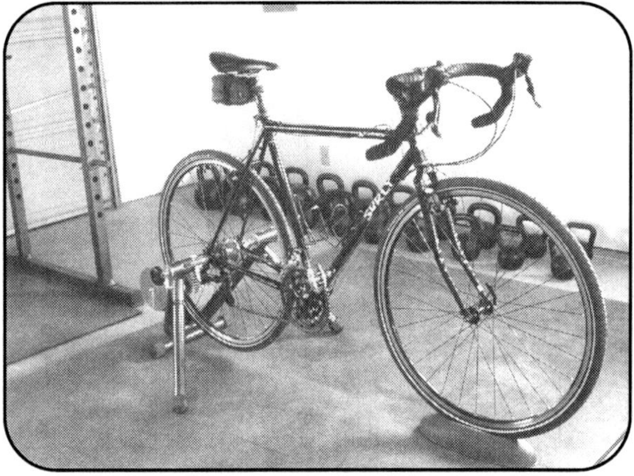

A bike trainer turns your bike into an effective indoor cardio training tool.

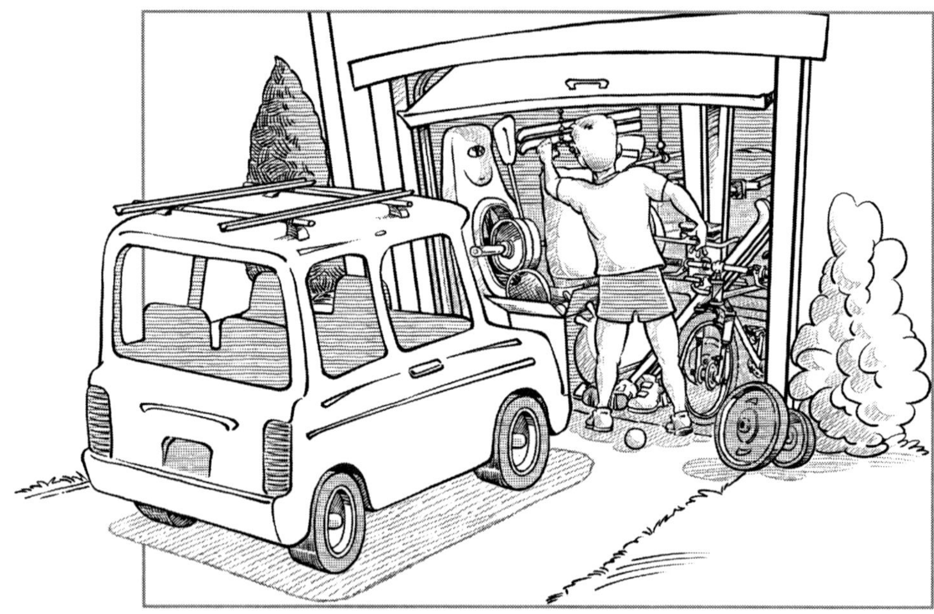

A garage full of gear equals a lot of fitness and fun – if it's used.

a real mess. A trainer with a large, heavy (at least three or four pound) flywheel will have a smoother more realistic road feel.

A high quality trainer will last for years. And a good one can help you stay super consistent with your cardio training, which makes this another must-have training tool.

A final word about equipment

All of the stuff listed above may seem like a lot, but it isn't, really. Just ask anyone who is serious about a sport, game, or hobby. A serious gearhead will have much more than the basics.

As you start and work into your strength and conditioning program also start to acquire the equipment you need. You will accumulate a wide variety of equipment that really works to improve your strength and conditioning. Remember to look for the best quality. It won't be long before your toolbox is complete.

10 Goals, Commitment, Motivation

One of the hardest parts of attaining and maintaining extraordinary fitness at any age is *consistency*. Yes, the workouts can be physically tough, but the hardest thing is having to do them week after week after week. That just wears on you mentally. This is especially true if you think of strength and conditioning training as "exercising" or "working out"—another chore to add to your already packed week. A painful, boring, slogging chore.

> Remember, fitness is what gives you the readiness and capability for whatever activity you choose.

You need to change your perspective and think of your workouts it as *training*. Training as an athlete. Developing skills and fitness in a fun and exciting way with the ultimate payoff being the ability to do some sport or activity. This athletic mindset can go a long way to helping you look forward to your strength and conditioning sessions.

Remember, fitness is what gives you the readiness and capability for whatever activity you choose.

To be successful in gaining fitness, four steps are absolutely vital. First, you have to honestly evaluate yourself and define your current level of fitness. Second, you need to set goals. Third, outline what you're going to do to reach your strength, cardio, and muscular endurance goals. The fourth and most important step is to put in your time. Ultimately, *fitness is the result of what you do*. It's the work you accomplish, not what you think or plan or feel. This four-step process is your way forward to successfully improving your strength and conditioning.

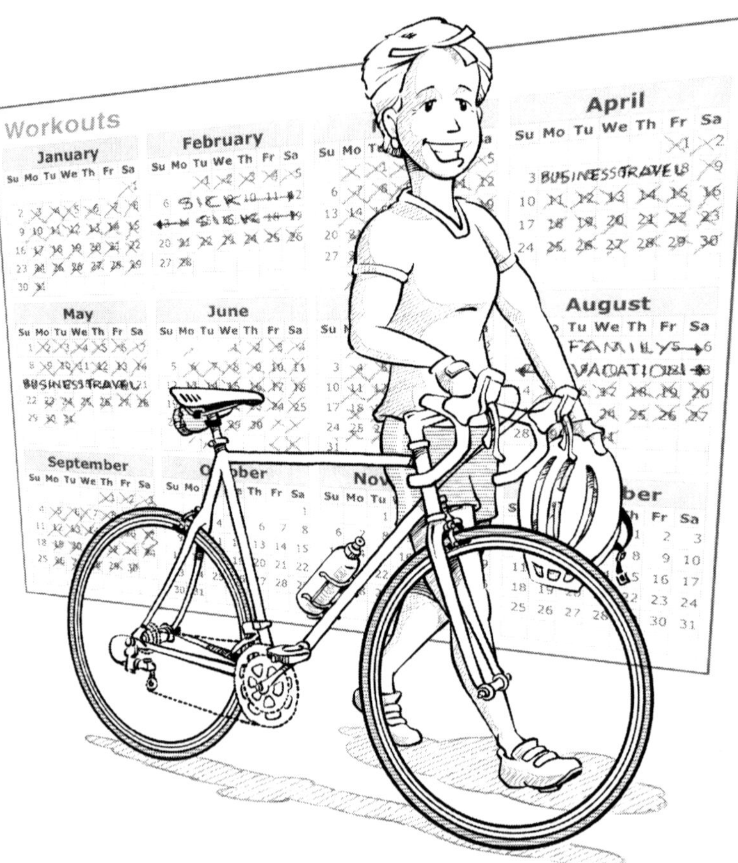

Consistency is vital to achieving and maintaining fitness.

But many people get stuck in this process long before they reach step four, taking action. There's so much information available on how to exercise that they get overwhelmed and confused. It's easier to sit there and be a couch potato than to try to figure out what to do to get fit.

That's why we've given specific recommendations on how to achieve high levels of strength and conditioning. Our recommendations aren't the only way to achieve this goal, of course. There are many other paths, many of which will also work. Our goal is to give a simple and effective path to help people achieve their fitness goals.

Evaluate your current fitness

When you evaluate your current level of fitness, the most important thing is to be honest with yourself. If your physical activity for the past few years was mostly sitting (in your car, in front of your computer, in front of your television), don't pretend that you're in "great" shape. If you've been exercising, but with low intensity by walking a treadmill while watching TV and/or lifting light, unchallenging weights, it's likely you're in better shape than the couch potato, but you're also not in "great" shape.

And, really, terms like "poor," "good" and "great" are subjective and essentially meaningless. So how do you accurately and honestly evaluate your current physical condition? The answer is testing. You need to physically test your strength, cardio condition, and muscular endurance. Testing will give you numbers that will pinpoint your current fitness.

Don't judge your test results. Don't apply terms like "poor," "good," or "great" to yourself. Your test results are just numbers that tell you where you are. Other people may have numbers higher or lower than yours, but that's not relevant. The relevant thing is to determine what your level of fitness is at this point in time. That's all.

We've given you some standards as guideposts. But use them to set upward goals, not to beat yourself down.

> How do you accurately and honestly evaluate your current physical condition? Testing will give you numbers that will pinpoint your current fitness.

We've explained how to test the three components of your fitness. To test your strength, determine how much weight you can lift for five reps in the Sumo deadlift and one arm kettlebell press. It's also a good idea to determine your five-rep maximum weight in the kettlebell front squat and to find out how many chin-ups you can do. Write down the results of this testing, which will accurately identify your current level of strength.

To test your cardio conditioning, take your power meter-equipped bike out for a ride and ride as hard as you can for eight minutes. Then on your next ride, ride as hard as you can for twenty minutes. Your average powers for those two efforts will pinpoint the current state of your cardio conditioning.

To test your level of muscular endurance, take a kettlebell that you can swing for sets of 20 repetitions and find out how many sets of 20 reps you can do at a pace of 36 seconds for each set of 20 reps with 36 seconds of rest in between. That will show you the level of your muscular endurance.

Obviously, you don't want to do this testing "cold" before you learn the exercises and become comfortable performing them. First, that could be dangerous. Pushing yourself while doing unfamiliar exercises isn't smart. Second, if you test using unfamiliar exercises, the results will not be an accurate reflection of your fitness. So spend some time learning the four strength exercises (Sumo deadlift, one-arm kettlebell press, kettlebell front squat, and chin-ups). Master the kettlebell swing. Ride your bike until it feels natural and learn how that power meter works. Then test yourself.

Now you have starting points. You know your current numbers and can work to improve them. They aren't subjective. They are accurate reflections of your current fitness. Now you can set some goals, develop an exercise plan, and start seriously working out. And then you can retest and accurately measure your progress in improving your strength and conditioning.

Set goals

When you set your goals, be sure to set behavior goals, not outcome goals. What's the difference? An example of a behavior goal is, "For the next two months, I'll do four weightlifting sessions a week." An outcome goal is, "In two months I'll win first place in my weight and age class at the Nevada State Powerlifting Championship."

What's the difference? You can control whether or not you succeed in reaching a behavior goal. You can control whether or not you do four weightlifting sessions every week. But you can't control the factors that determine whether you'll achieve an outcome goal. You can't count on becoming the best weightlifter in Nevada.

Another example of an outcome goal that you can't count on achieving would be increasing your 20-minute bicycling power by 10 percent in the next seven weeks. Whether or not you achieve this goal depends on factors that you can't control. Factors such as your genetic ability to improve your cardio conditioning and your current level of fitness. If your fitness level is already high, it's much harder to make large further improvement, whereas if your fitness level is low, it's much easier to make large improvement. Set a behavior goal instead. This can be riding four times a week with 40 to 60 minutes of intervals and reaching 350 TSS points for five of the next seven weeks and reaching 175 TSS points for two of those weeks.

> To make your goals real, you need to write them down. You absolutely must keep a workout log.

Setting behavior goals doesn't mean that you ignore outcomes. It's appropriate to test the outcomes of what you do to reach your goals. You do this by retesting your strength, cardio condition, and muscular endurance on a regular basis. In fact, we encourage you to keep careful track of test outcomes, like being able to lift heavier weights, increasing your bicycling power levels, and increasing the number of kettlebell swing sets you can do. Seeing progress over time is tremendously motivating. It can really help you stay consistent with your strength and conditioning training.

To make your goals real, you need to write them down. Write them on the front cover of a small notebook. Then record your workouts in the notebook and review your progress at least once a week to make sure that you're moving toward your goals. You absolutely must keep a workout log. Nobody's memory is good enough to track what you've been doing for long periods of time . . . not to mention that it's easy to selectively remember what you did or didn't do. In a workout log, it's there in black and white.

A more positive function of a training log is that it shows you your progress. You know when you reach each goal. This can be immensely helpful in keeping you motivated with your strength and conditioning program.

Let's face facts—effective exercise can be boring. Doing the exercises and workouts in this book can become tedious. Most people want variety. Our question to you is this: *Do you want entertainment or do you want results?*

We suggest that you use the techniques in this book to get really fit and entertain yourself by using your fitness. Go hiking, mountain climbing, skiing, scuba diving, kayaking. Your choices to use and exhibit your physical capabilities are endless.

You can also set goals for a competition—a weightlifting meet, bike race, or kettlebell competition. This can create intense focus and give you an opportunity to really push yourself and see what you're capable of achieving. Get involved. Whatever your age, become a competitive athlete. There are master's competitions for almost every sport. Becoming an athlete can help you stay motivated.

Some people complain that it's too hard. The flippant answer is that it has to be hard. Without intensity, you can't increase your fitness. The real answer is that if it's truly too hard, then you need to start easier and work up over time. Appropriate exercise is never too hard. This is a topic we'll deal with in greater detail in the next chapter.

But maybe the real problem here is one of low expectations. After reading about lifting heavy weights, VO2 max intervals done on the bicycle, or swinging kettlebells, you may be saying to yourself, "There's no way I can do all that." Well, we believe you're more capable than you think you are. Take on the challenge. You'll make progress and improve your physical fitness. Probably your mental fitness, too.

> We suggest that you use the techniques in this book to get really fit and entertain yourself by using your fitness. Go hiking, mountain climbing, skiing, scuba diving, kayaking. Your choices to use and exhibit your physical capabilities are endless.

Outline your fitness program

If you set appropriate behavior goals in each of the three components of fitness, outlining your fitness program is done. That's because your goals will set out precisely what you're going to do in the coming weeks to work on your strength, cardio conditioning, and muscular endurance.

Do it!

Now comes the final and most important step—taking action. You must do the work to meet the goals you set. There should be no doubt in your mind that you can achieve those goals. And when you do the work and reach your goals, the results will follow. Again, there should be no doubt that if you achieve your goals, results will follow. You will become stronger. You will gain greater endurance and cardiovascular health. You will become leaner and more muscular.

So that's the process. But following through with that process—setting goals, being committed, and staying motivated—must, in the final analysis, come from within you. This is what is called intrinsic motivation. Extrinsic motivation comes from outside of you. Your wife telling you that you need to get in shape is extrinsic motivation. You telling yourself is intrinsic motivation. Extrinsic motivators may get you started, but they tend to peter out. Another example of extrinsic motivation is winning in a sport. Extrinsic motivation might lead you to success, but success is about having, which implies you can lose it and is always temporary.

> You must do the work to meet the goals you set. There should be no doubt in your mind that you can achieve those goals.

Long-term commitment requires intrinsic motivation. It's about excellence in terms of being the best that you can be. Being who you are is permanent. You can't lose it. If you see yourself as an athlete, and that becomes your being, then staying committed to your strength and conditioning training is easy because it's a natural part of who you are.

11

Finding Your Own Way to Extraordinary Fitness

We've presented the core principles of our training techniques and programs and made recommendations as to how to implement those principles. Now, as you start your personal journey to extraordinary fitness, it's your turn to do some thinking and planning.

It's all about strength and conditioning. It's about complete fitness that includes strength, cardio conditioning, and muscular endurance. It's about customizing your workouts to your life. Most likely, you'll fall into one of three groups.

Group one consists of multi-sport master's athletes and the very active. These athletes are strong and in great shape, both cardio-wise and muscular endurance-wise. This very small group can use the principles presented in this book to improve and simplify their basic strength and conditioning training.

Group two consists of active individuals, like runners who are in good shape in a single aspect of strength and conditioning but not all three aspects. Runners tend to be fit cardio-wise, but weak and with poor body composition (low muscle mass).

Then there is group three. This is the "I want to be fit" group. People who are currently lacking in all three areas of strength and conditioning.

Start by thinking about which group you're in right now. What are your strengths and weaknesses? Your preferences? Think hard about what you need to do to get more fit. If you participate in sports, how will you fit a strength and conditioning program with doing your sport?

If you're overweight, how are you going to proceed?

If you haven't been doing strength and conditioning, or only doing some of the work, you need to start now and proceed in a slow and deliberate manner.

No matter which group you're in, starting out for everyone involves slowly building up all three elements of strength and conditioning: strength, cardio endurance, and muscular endurance. Always start easy. Slowly work into the full program described in the previous chapters.

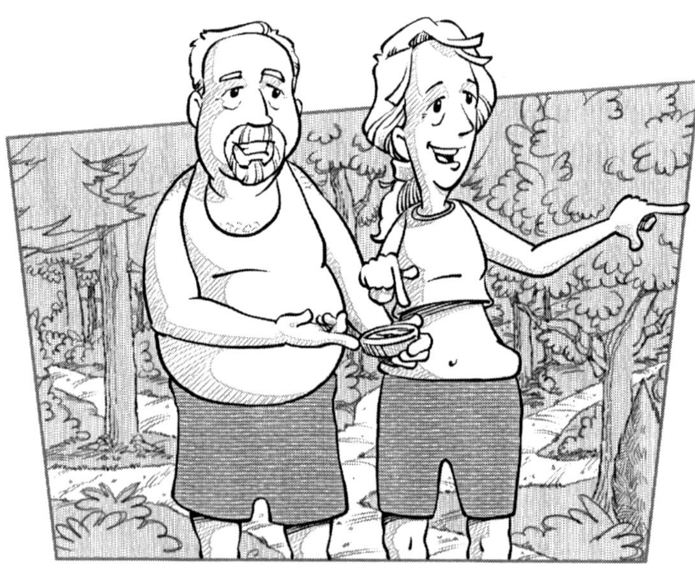

Now we're headed in the right direction!

We've given you a straightforward program that works. Very few of you will be able to jump into the full program. You'll need to work into the full program over many months.

So let's talk more about starting out in each of the three areas and then moving into all three areas together. You will need to start by picking the one area that you most need or want to focus on. This can be strength or cardio conditioning or muscular endurance conditioning. Get started. Slowly build into the full program for that area. In the beginning, you can ignore the other two areas.

Starting out developing your cardio conditioning

For example, when you start with cardio conditioning, you can start by working up to riding your bike four times a week. In the beginning, don't do any intervals. Just ride four days a week, working up to about an hour of riding each day. Once this is comfortable, test your power at VO2 max and your power at LT. Then start to add intervals to your weekly rides. Start with one eight-minute 30:30 VO2 max interval, or one eight-minute LT interval, or one eight-minute combo interval as your hard day for the week. For your other three rides each week, just keep riding. Then move to two intervals on your hard day and one on your easy days. Mix up the intervals, but make sure to do some VO2 max work every week. As you build up your cardio endurance over the next weeks, add intervals to both your hard and easy rides until you're doing four intervals on your hard day and two intervals on your easy days. Track your heart rate during the intervals, and when it's consistently lower than before, retest your power at VO2 max and at LT. Then reset your interval power levels. This process will most likely take two or three months or more. Usually it's best to move on to strength or muscular endurance work, even if you haven't worked up to the full cardio program. You can do that when you rotate back later.

However far you've gotten in your cardio training after one to three months, put it in maintenance mode and move on to either strength or muscular endurance training.

Starting out increasing your strength

When you're starting strength training again, start slowly. Start with a couple of sessions a week in which you're learning how to do the lifts properly, experimenting with ladders, and finding the weights that you feel comfortable using. Then start using ladders on the deadlift and overhead press twice a week. Make both workouts easy at first. Then make one session hard and the other easy. Over the next weeks, add one or two more easy sessions every week.

As you get stronger, increase the weights in both exercises. But always keep the increases moderate (three to five percent). Like cardio conditioning, this may well take more than three months. Don't stress about that. You'll get to the full program soon enough.

Starting out building your muscular endurance

When you begin muscular endurance training, at first just do kettlebell swings. Leave the snatching and cleaning and jerking for the future. As with strength training, start easy twice a week, working easily and building up the number of reps per set and sets that you're doing, always stretching just a bit outside your comfort zone. Over the weeks, make one session each week your hard session, in which you swing longer and one session easier in which you swing less. Then add one or two more easy sessions for a total of three or four sessions a week. Remember that the goal is to swing more until you reach 21 to 35 sets during your hard workouts.

After two or three months, no matter how much progress you've made, switch back to a cardio or strength focus. Remember that as you move out of a focus period, you're switching to maintenance. You're moving from the cardio focus period to a strength focus with a cardio maintenance period. Then you can move to a muscular endurance focus with cardio and strength maintenance periods.

You've achieved a complete fitness program!

As you've slowly worked into each area, you've also now worked into the complete program. Depending on your starting condition, this may take months or even years. Remember—*there's no rush. You're only competing against yourself.* It's very important that you work into the program this way so as not be become overwhelmed physically and/or mentally.

Once you've worked into the full program, you'll have a results-driven routine (your exercise program), which can then be used for enjoyment-driven recreational activities and that has major side benefits like better health and functionality in all areas of your life.

> Remember—*there's no rush. You're only competing against yourself.* It's very important that you work into the program this way so as not be become overwhelmed physically and/or mentally.

Coordinating your fitness program with your sport(s)

But what if you're already an athlete? What if you're really into one or more sports? If you play softball, basketball, soccer, or tennis, or compete in running, swimming, triathlon, or skiing, or you're serious about some other sport, how do you schedule the time it takes to develop your sports skills plus develop your strength and conditioning?

As we said earlier, improving all aspects of strength and conditioning at the same time is just not possible. Similarly, improving your strength and conditioning and improving sports skills at the same time is also pretty much impossible.

The solution is to designate an in-season and an off-season over the course of a year. In your off-season, spend your time improving the various facets of your strength and conditioning and do just a minimum of work to maintain your sports skills. During your in-season, focus on your sport and put your strength and conditioning work into maintenance mode. What is maintenance mode? On two days of the week, do some cardio, and on another two days, do a combined strength and muscular endurance workout. This is six short sessions a week spread over four days a week. That's it. The rest of the time is open for the specific exercises and workouts of your sport.

You may have to create artificial seasons for yourself. For example, tennis is a year-round sport in Southern California. You might play a spring season and a fall season for several months each. That makes summer and winter your strength and conditioning seasons.

This full maintenance program is appropriate for many sports, such as soccer, skiing, and tennis, that require integrated strength, conditioning, and muscular endurance. There are sports that emphasize one area, and if you play one of those, you'll need to change to a partial maintenance plan. For example, if your sport is bicycle racing or triathlon, you will be working your cardio fitness to the max, so there's no point in doing maintenance for cardio in your strength and conditioning program. Just do strength and muscular endurance maintenance work. Another example is powerlifting. If you compete in this sport, which tests your maximum strength, there is no need for strength maintenance work. Just do cardio and some muscular endurance training.

What to do when life happens

A maintenance phase is also very useful for the times of the year when other demands on your time are particularly time-consuming. If you're a CPA, tax season from January to April is crazy. Go into a maintenance program during tax season and return to a full program after April 15. You shouldn't lose much, if any, fitness, and you can pick up again where you left off. The key is to make time for the short maintenance routine. Just don't blow off exercise altogether.

This book gives you the general principles and teaches you how to reach extraordinary levels of strength and conditioning. Now it's up to you to tailor what you've learned into a program that will work for you and will fit in with your life.

Much of what we've presented is not conventional wisdom. You may have some skepticism. But try implementing these principles of effective strength and conditioning training that we've presented to you in this book. See for yourself that these principles do work.

Final Thoughts on Staying Fit in Real Life

Working to achieve extraordinary levels of strength and conditioning is a lifelong pursuit that will have its ups and downs.

This book deals with general principles, not hard and fast rules or rigid schedules. Rules and/or rigid schedules are hard to follow; principles are softer. You can cut yourself some slack. If you follow the principles, results will follow. Seeing results helps prevent you from getting discouraged because you broke this or that rule or missed a scheduled workout. Results also help you stay consistent in your workouts.

Consistency is what it's all about. You need to keep going and going and going. It's not fair, but if you stop you will regress and eventually lose your fitness. As we get older, consistency becomes even more vital because gaining fitness becomes harder, while losing it becomes a whole lot easier. This need for consistency is the hardest thing to deal with. It truly wears on you. Competition and other motivational techniques can help with consistency, but in the end it comes down to self-mastery. Don't wait for motivation to come to you. Just do it.

> Working to achieve extraordinary levels of strength and conditioning is a lifelong pursuit that will have its ups and downs.

Our bodies are constantly changing, which is another reason you need to be both consistent and flexible. At different times your focus can be on different things. As long as you continue to follow the basic principles, you'll be OK. And, yes, life does tend to throw us curve balls that we need to work through. Sickness, accidents, grief, money woes … the list is endless. You'll find that consistent exercise can help you work through these things. Or you can use them as an excuse to quit. Quitting is easy. Consistency is hard. And consistency also becomes harder as you get older. You take on additional responsibilities in your life that leave you with less time. You find that gaining fitness is more difficult and takes longer, while losing fitness is easy and happens more quickly. It seems like you're fighting a losing battle with rust.

Yes, reaching and keeping high levels of strength and conditioning when you're not as young as you used to be becomes a challenge. But meeting that challenge can be rewarding. Most of what we all consider to be "normal aging" is, in fact, just disuse. The reality is that with consistent exercise and a reasonable diet you can keep very high levels of strength and conditioning well into your 70s. You can be as functional at 80 as you were at 50!

> Reaching and keeping high levels of strength and conditioning when you're not as young as you used to be becomes a challenge. But meeting that challenge can be rewarding. Most of what we all consider to be "normal aging" is, in fact, just disuse. The reality is that with consistent exercise and a reasonable diet you can keep very high levels of strength and conditioning well into your 70s.

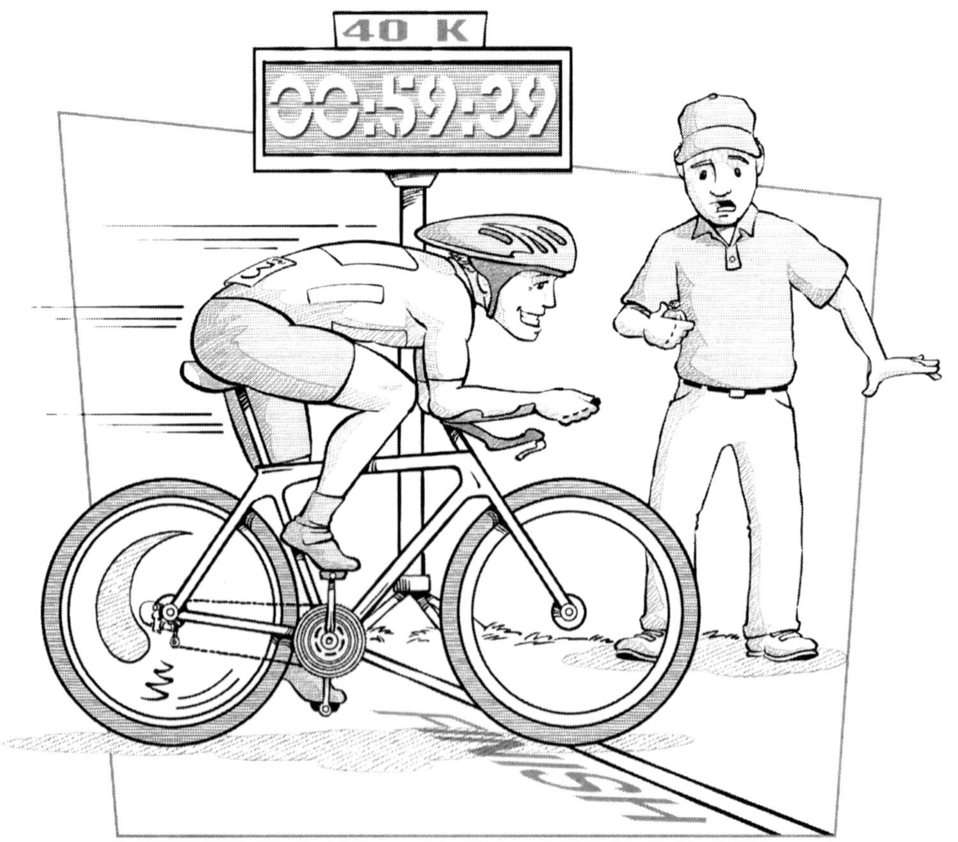

Age isn't a barrier to great physical performance.

This flies in the face of conventional wisdom, but master's athletes in all sports are proving that it can be done. Having crossed the age 50 milestone, both Andy and Michelle can honestly say that we're in better physical condition than we were in our twenties. And our athletic performances in bicycling and powerlifting are also better. And we see other athletes 10, 20, or more years older than we are still competing at very high levels in powerlifting and bicycling. They pull off performances that most people find unbelievable. They're the result of consistent intense exercise coupled with enough time for recovery and a good diet.

And long-term intense exercise has been shown to slow cellular aging by reducing the shortening of telomeres that occurs with aging. Intense exercise also stimulates your body to produce lots of mitochondria, which are the power source of the cells in your body. The more mitochondria a cell has, the more energy available to it to perform whatever functions that it's designed to. With increased fitness, your cells are healthier and you can enjoy a longer as well as a much more functional life. What could be a better reason to strive for super strength, and conditioning?

Our wish for every reader, whatever your age or situation, is that you become an athlete and internalize strength and conditioning into your being, into who you are. And that by becoming an athlete, you train consistently and pursue excellence in strength and conditioning for the rest of your life.

What are telomeres? Telomeres are the "end caps" on the chromosomes in your cells. As cells divide over time, the telomeres get shorter. The hypothesis is that as our telomeres shorten, our chromosomes no longer work properly. The result is that the cells age and eventually become senescent. Telomeres are affected by environmental factors. Stress, for example, can cause them to shorten more quickly. In contrast, exercise has been shown to maintain telomere length. When the telomeres stay long, our cells will have a longer lifespan and, at least in theory, we will, too.

Glossary

Acute training load (ATL) – A measure of the physical stress and the level of fatigue currently being experienced by your body due to your exercise workload over the most recent seven days.

Aerobic – With oxygen. Refers to your body's ability to process and use oxygen to do its work.

Aerobic capacity – How long you can go at a percentage of your VO2 max. A measure of the endurance capabilities of your body.

Aerobic speed – The maximum sustained speed that you can go powered by your heart, lungs, and circulatory system.

Anabolic – Refers to your body's metabolic processes that use energy to build up its organs and tissues. Building larger muscles is an anabolic process.

Anabolic burst – Manipulating your diet and exercise program to change your body composition noticeably in a short period of time. Accelerating the anabolic process of building muscle by using energy from stored fat deposits.

Beta-alanine – A supplement that is an amino acid that increases carnosine levels in your muscles. Muscles with higher levels of carnosine are stronger and have greater endurance.

Body recomposition – The process of building muscle and losing fat so that you become leaner and more muscular.

Body-mass index (BMI) – An index that uses height and weight to determine whether someone is underweight, normal weight, overweight, or obese. It is of limited usefulness because is based on body weight, not body composition.

Cardio training – Exercises that stress your central cardiovascular system (heart, lungs, and circulatory system). These are exercises that are done on a continuous basis, like cycling, running, swimming, cross-country skiing, etc.

Cardiovascular capacity (VO2 max) – The maximum amount of oxygen your heart and lungs can take in and distribute throughout your body. VO2 max is measured in milliliters of oxygen used per minute per kilogram of body weight. It is a measure of the capability of your central cardiovascular system.

Chronic training load (CTL) – A measure of your level of fitness and ability to perform physically as a result of the amount of exercise you've done in the past seven weeks.

Clean – A weightlifting exercise in which you pull a barbell, dumbbell, or kettlebell up off the floor and guide it to a racked position on your shoulders. It can be done as a standalone exercise or combined with another exercise like a press or a jerk to become a clean and press or clean and jerk.

Coenzyme Q (COQ) – A vital substance that fuels the mitochondria in all of your body's cells. In the mitochondria, COQ aids in the conversion of food into energy that powers cell functions. A supplement that works to make sure your cells have sufficient energy to function properly. Muscle and heart cells that have sufficient Coenzyme Q are stronger and have greater endurance.

Combination (combo) interval – An interval that combines a VO2 max interval with a lactate threshold (LT) interval. It trains both your cardiovascular capacity and endurance.

Concentrated carbohydrates – Starch and sugar that come in the form of grains, beans, potatoes, dairy products, sugar, honey, and fruit juices. You need to avoid these foods except after an intense workout.

Conditioning – The process of developing your body's aerobic capabilities. Includes improving the capacity of your central cardiovascular system as well as increasing your muscular endurance.

Creatine Monohydrate – A supplement that works by helping your muscle cells absorb water. Fully hydrated muscles cells work more efficiently and as a consequence are stronger.

Criterium – A Latin word that means "circuit" used to describe a bicycle race of many laps around the same course. Bike racing is a Eurocentric sport, so here in the U.S. we also call bicycle circuit races criteriums

Daily singles – A method of strength training that can be used for short periods of time to quickly boost your level of strength. Involves lifting heavy weights for many sets of one rep.

Electrolytes – Elements that your body requires to function properly. They include sodium, potassium, magnesium, and calcium. Heavy sweating due to intense exercise or heat or both depletes your body's electrolytes, and you need to replace them from sources in your diet.

Five-count pedaling –A pedaling technique that involves counting your pedal strokes and pushing hard on some and easing up on others. Works to reduce muscular fatigue in your legs, enabling you to pedal harder and longer.

Glycogen – A form of carbohydrate that your body stores in your muscles and liver so that energy can be quickly available for intense efforts.

Indoor trainer – A device you attach your bicycle to that converts it into a stationary bike that can be ridden indoors. That way, you can use the same bike for both outdoor and indoor riding.

Insulin – An important body hormone that is involved in storing fat. Excess insulin is associated with obesity and Type 2 diabetes. To be lean and healthy, it is important to control your insulin levels. This is best accomplished by controlling what, when and how much you eat.

Joint mobility - The ability of your joints to move smoothly through a full range of motion.

Kcal – Kilocalories. A measure of the energy content of food.

Lactate threshold (LT) – The percentage of your VO2 max that you can sustain for a longer period of time, usually defined as one hour. A measure of the endurance capability of your aerobic system.

Muscular endurance – The ability of your muscles generate a high muscular workload for an extended period of time. The muscular part of conditioning. Also, a critical part of becoming lean and muscular because muscular endurance training builds muscles and reduces fat stores.

Paleo diet – The diet of our hunter-gatherer ancestors. This is the diet that humans evolved to function best on. In a nutshell—*do eat* meats and fish, vegetables, nuts, berries, and fruits. *Don't eat* grains, beans, potatoes, dairy, and sugar.

Rep ladders – The most efficient and effective method of increasing your strength. Involves lifting heavy weights in only a few exercises using a 1-2-3-1-2-3-1-2-3 rep pattern.

Reserve capacity – The difference between your resting heart rate and maximum heart rate. Gives your heart the ability to respond to stress without breaking down.

Spinning – A popular method of cardio exercise involving riding an indoor fixed gear bicycle following the lead of an instructor who has you do intervals by having you alternately pedal harder and faster, then slower and easier.

Taper - In terms of athletic competition, "taper" has a very specific meaning. It's a part of preparing for and event or competition and refers to changing your training for a week or two before an event so that on the day of the event you're fresh (not fatigued) and still have a high level of fitness.

Telomeres – The "end caps" on the chromosomes in your body's cells. As cells divide over time, the telomeres shorten, which causes the cells to age and eventually become senescent. Exercise has been shown to maintain telomere length and extend the healthy life of cells. In theory, this extends our healthy lives, too.

Tempo or hard-endurance pace – When doing cardio conditioning training, your tempo pace is 90 percent of your LT pace. This is a pace that will increase your cardio endurance.

Training stress balance (TSB) – This is the difference between your chronic training load (CTL) and your acute training load (ATL). TSB = CTL – ATL. It provides insight into your levels of fitness and fatigue.

Training stress score (TSS) – This score combines the intensity and volume of your bicycle rides and provides a number that quantifies the stress that that level of intensity and volume puts on your body.

Bibliography

Chapter 1

Bass, Clarence. *Challenge Yourself At Any Age: A Guide to Intelligent Training by the Foremost Proponent of the All-Round Fitness Lifestyle.* Clarence Bass' Ripped Enterprises, 1999.

Bergquist, Lee. *Second Wind: The Rise of the Ageless Athlete.* Human Kinetics, 2009.

Mayhew, Ed. *Fitter After 50: Forever Changing Our Beliefs about Aging.* 1st Books Library, 2002.

Chapter 2

Bompa, Tudor. *Periodization of Strength: The New Wave in Strength Training.* Veritas Publishing Inc., 1993.

Bompa, Tudor and Cornacchia, Lorenzo. *Serious Strength Training: Periodization for building muscle power and mass.* Human Kinetics, 1998.

Drechsler, Arthur. *The Weightlifting Encyclopedia: A Guide to World Class Performance.* A is A Communications, 1998.

Everett, Greg. *Olympic Weightlifting: A Complete Guide for Athletes & Coaches.* Catalyst Athletics, LLC, 2008.

Frantz, Ernie. *Ernie Frantz's Ten Commandments of Powerlifting.* Darwill Press, no date.

Gallagher, Marty. *Coan: The Man, The Myth, The Method.* Coan Quest, Inc, 1999.

———. *The Purposeful Primitive: From Fat and Flaccid to Lean and Powerful.* Dragon Door Publications, 2008.

Justa, Steve. *Rock Iron Steel: The Book of Strength.* IronMind Enterprises, Inc., 1998.

McRobert, Stuart. *Beyond Brawn: The Insider's encyclopedia on How To Build Muscle & Might.* CS Publishing Ltd., 1998.

Newton, Harvey. *Explosive Lifting for Sports: Boost power with the snatch, clean, jerk, squat and other dynamic lifts.* Human Kinetics, 2002.

O'Shea, Patrick. *Quantum Strength & Power Training (Gaining the Winning Edge): Textbook of Applied Athletic Strength Training & Conditioning for Peak Performance Ages 16-80.* Patrick's Books, 1996.

Poliquin, Charles. *German Body Comp Program: Burn fat and build muscle with the only program that uses weight training for weight loss.* Poliquin Performance Centers, 2004.

———. *The Poliquin Principles: Successful Methods for Strength and Mass Development.* Dayton Writers Group, 1997.

Sisco, Peter and Little, John. *Power Factor Training: A Scientific Approach to Building Lean Muscle Mass.* Contemporary Books, 1997.

Staley, Charles. *Muscle Logic: Escalating Density Training Changes the Rules for Maximum-Impact Weight Training.* Rodale, 2005.

Starr, Bill. *The Strongest Shall Survive: Strength Training for Football.* Fitness Consultants and Supply, 1996.

Tsatsouline, Pavel. *Beyond Bodybuilding: Muscle and Strength Training Secrets for the Renaissance Man.* Dragon Door Publications, 2005.

———. *The Naked Warrior: Master the Secrets of the Super-Strong-Using Bodyweight Exercises Only.* Dragon Door Publications, 2003.

———. *Power to the People! Russian Strength Training Secrets for Every American.* Dragon Door Publications, 1999.

———. *Power to the People Professional: How to Add 100s of Pounds to Your Squat, Bench, and Deadlift With Advanced Russian Techniques Russian Strength Training Secrets for Every American.* Dragon Door Publications, 2009.

Chapter 3

Allen, Hunter and Coggan, Andrew. *Training and Racing With a Power Meter (2nd edition).* Velopress, 2010.

Armstrong, Lance and Carmichael, Chris. *The Lance Armstrong Performance Program; 7 Weeks to the Perfect Ride.* Rodale, 2000.

Baker, Arnie. *Smart Cycling: Successful Training & Racing for Riders of All Levels.* Argo Publishing, 1996.

Borysewicz, Edward. *Bicycle Road Racing: Complete Program for Training and Competition.* Vitesse Press, 1985.

Burke, Edmund. *Serious Cycling (2nd Edition).* Human Kinetics, 2002.

Carmichael, Chris and Rutberg, Jim. *The Time-crunched Cyclist: Fit, Fast, and Powerfuls in 6 Hours a Week.* Velopress, 2009.

———. *The Ultimate Ride: Get Fit, Get Fast, and Start Winning with the World's Top Cycling Coach.* G.P. Putnam's Sons, 2003.

Friel, Joe. *Cycling Past 50: For fitness and performance through the years.* Human Kinetics, 1998.

———. *The Cyclist's Training Bible (3rd Edition).* VeloPress, 2003.

———. *The Mountain Biker's Training Bible.* VeloPress, 2000.

Janssen, Peter. *Lactate Threshold Training.* Human Kinetics, 2001.

Jeukendrup, Asker. *High Performance Cycling.* Human Kinetics, 2002.

LeMond, Greg and Gordis, Kent. *Greg LeMond's Complete Book of Bicycling.* The Putnam Publishing Group, 1987.

Niles, Rick. *Time-Saving Training for Multisport Athletes: How to Fit Workouts into Work Days.* Human Kinetics, 1997.

Phinney, Davis and Carpenter, Connie. *Training For Cycling: The Ultimate Guide to Improved Performance.* The Berkley Publishing Group, 1992.

Ross, Michael. *Maximum Performance for Cyclists.* Velopress, 2005.

Chapter 4

Jay, Kenneth. *Viking Warrior Conditioning: The Scientific Approach to Forging a Heart of Elastic Steel – An Application of the Theory Behind Proper VO2 Max Training.* Dragon Door Publications, 2009.

Tsatsouline, Pavel. *Enter the Kettlebell: Strength Secret of the Soviet Supermen.* Dragon Door Publications, 2006.

———. *From Russia with Tough Love: Pavel's Kettlebell Workout for a Femme Fatale.* Dragon Door Publications, 2002.

———. *Return of the Kettlebell: Explosive Kettlebell Training for Explosive Muscle Gains.* Dragon Door Publications, 2009.

———. *The Russian Kettlebell Challenge: Xtreme Fitness for Hard Living Comrades.* Dragon Door Publications, 2001.

Schwartz, Leonard. *The Heavyhands Walking Book! An Open Invitation to Convert Walking into a Lifelong Total Fitness Strategy.* Panaerobics Press, 1990.

Chapter 7

Audette, Ray. *Neanderthin: Eat Like a Caveman to Achieve a Lean, Strong, Healthy Body.* St. Martin's Press, 1999.

Cordain, Loren. *The Paleo Diet: Lose Weight and Get Healthy by Eating the Food You Were Designed to Eat.* John Wiley & Sons, Inc., 2002.

Cordain, Loren and Friel, Joe. *The Paleo Diet for Athletes: A Nutritional Formula for Peak Athletic Performance.* Rodale, 2005.

Hofmekler, Ori. *The Warrior Diet: How to Take Advantage of Undereating and Overeating.* Dragon Door Publications, 2001.

Schmid, Ronald. *Native Nutrition: Eating According to Ancestral Wisdom.* Healing Arts Press, 1994.

Chapter 8

Tsatsouline, Pavel. *Beyond Stretching: Russian Flexibility Breakthroughs.* Dragon Door Publications, 1998.

———. *Relax into Stretch: Instant Flexibility Through Mastering Muscle Tension.* Dragon Door Publications, 2001.

———. *Super Joints: Russian Longevity Secrets for Pain-Free Movement, Maximum Mobility & Flexible Strength.* Dragon Door Publications, 2001.

Index

N

O

P

CPSIA information can be obtained at www.ICGtesting.com
Printed in the USA
BVOW052359041012

302157BV00003B/1/P